THE COMPREHENSIVE DMSO HEALING GUIDE [20 IN 1]

The Ultimate Science-Backed Solution to Erase Pain, Reduce Inflammation, Restore Mobility and Regain Your Health Naturally

EMILY BRADFORD

© Copyright 2025 by (Emily Bradford) - All rights reserved.

This document is geared towards providing exact and reliable information regarding the topic and issue covered. The publication is sold with the idea that the publisher is not required to render accounting, officially permitted, or otherwise, qualified services. If advice is necessary, legal, or professional, a practiced individual in the profession should be ordered.

In no way is it legal to reproduce, duplicate, or transmit any part of this document in either electronic means or in printed format. Recording of this publication is strictly prohibited and any storage of this document is not allowed unless with written permission from the publisher. All rights reserved.

The information provided herein is stated to be truthful and consistent, in that any liability, in terms of inattention or otherwise, by any usage or abuse of any policies, processes, or directions contained within is the solitary and utter responsibility of the recipient reader. Under no circumstances will any legal responsibility or blame be held against the publisher for any reparation, damages, or monetary loss due to the information herein, either directly or indirectly.

Respective authors own all copyrights not held by the publisher.

The information herein is offered for informational purposes solely and is universal as so. The presentation of the information is without contract or any type of guaranteed assurance.

The trademarks that are used are without any consent, and the publication of the trademark is without permission or backing by the trademark owner. All trademarks and brands within this book are for clarifying purposes only and are owned by the owners themselves, not affiliated with this document.

TABLE OF CONTENTS

BOOK 1
THE SCIENCE BEHIND DMSO – UNDERSTANDING THE HEALING MOLECULE 11

CHAPTER 1
WHAT IS DMSO AND HOW DOES IT WORK? 13
The Unique Chemical Structure and Its Role in Healing 13
Why DMSO Is So Effective: A Deep Dive into Its Mechanism 15

CHAPTER 2
THE HISTORY AND MEDICAL EVOLUTION OF DMSO 17
From Industrial Solvent to Medical Marvel: The Journey of DMSO 17
Why Mainstream Medicine Overlooks DMSO: Regulations and Politics 18

BOOK 2
DMSO FOR CHRONIC PAIN RELIEF 21

CHAPTER 3
THE ROLE OF DMSO IN PAIN MANAGEMENT 23
How DMSO Blocks Pain Signals and Reduces Inflammation 23
Comparing DMSO to NSAIDs and Opioids: The Safer Alternative 24

CHAPTER 4
USING DMSO FOR ARTHRITIS, FIBROMYALGIA, AND NEUROPATHY 27
Targeting Joint Pain and Stiffness with DMSO Protocols 27
Healing Nerve Damage: DMSO for Neuropathy and Sciatica 28

BOOK 3
DMSO FOR INJURY RECOVERY AND POST-SURGICAL HEALING 31

CHAPTER 5
SPEEDING UP HEALING WITH DMSO 33
How DMSO Reduces Swelling and Bruising Post-Injury 33
Enhancing Tissue Repair: DMSO for Sprains, Strains, and Tears 34

CHAPTER 6
POST-SURGICAL RECOVERY AND SCAR REDUCTION 37
Reducing Adhesions and Scar Formation with DMSO 37
How DMSO Aids in Post-Surgical Inflammation Control 38

BOOK 4
THE ANTI-INFLAMMATORY POWER OF DMSO 41

CHAPTER 7
INFLAMMATION – THE ROOT OF CHRONIC DISEASE 43
Understanding Chronic Inflammation and Autoimmune Responses 43
How DMSO Neutralizes Inflammatory Cytokines and Free Radicals 44

CHAPTER 8
DMSO PROTOCOLS FOR INFLAMMATORY CONDITIONS 47
Treating Rheumatoid Arthritis, Tendonitis, and Gout 47
DMSO Combinations: Using MSM, Turmeric, and Omega-3s for Maximum Effect 49

BOOK 5
DMSO FOR JOINT AND MUSCLE HEALTH 51

CHAPTER 9
STRENGTHENING JOINTS AND PREVENTING DEGENERATION 53
Rebuilding Cartilage with DMSO and Supporting Nutrients 53
Long-Term Use of DMSO for Osteoarthritis Management 54

CHAPTER 10
DMSO FOR MUSCLE RECOVERY AND SPORTS INJURIES 57
Enhancing Athletic Performance and Recovery with DMSO 57
Treating Ligament and Tendon Damage for Faster Healing 58

BOOK 6
DMSO FOR SKIN CONDITIONS AND WOUND HEALING 61

CHAPTER 11
THE SKIN-REJUVENATING POWER OF DMSO 63
Treating Burns, Cuts, and Ulcers with DMSO Applications 63
Using DMSO for Chronic Skin Conditions: Eczema, Psoriasis, and Dermatitis 64

CHAPTER 12
ANTI-AGING AND COSMETIC BENEFITS OF DMSO 67
DIY DMSO-Based Skin Serums for a Youthful Glow 67
DIY DMSO-Based Skin Serums for a Youthful Glow 68

BOOK 7
DMSO FOR IMMUNE SUPPORT AND INFECTIONS 71

CHAPTER 13
FIGHTING BACTERIAL INFECTIONS WITH DMSO 73
Treating Staph, Cellulitis, and UTIs Naturally 73
Enhancing Antibiotic Efficacy with DMSO 74

CHAPTER 14
DMSO'S ROLE IN VIRAL AND FUNGAL INFECTIONS 77
Using DMSO for Herpes, Shingles, and Respiratory Viruses 77
Treating Candida and Other Fungal Overgrowths 79

BOOK 8
DMSO FOR AUTOIMMUNE DISORDERS 81

CHAPTER 15
BALANCING THE IMMUNE SYSTEM WITH DMSO 83
How DMSO Regulates Overactive Immune Responses 83
Managing Autoimmune Conditions Like Lupus and MS 84

CHAPTER 16
DMSO FOR THYROID HEALTH 87
Supporting Hashimoto's and Hypothyroidism with DMSO 87
DMSO and Selenium: A Powerful Anti-Inflammatory Duo 88

BOOK 9
DMSO FOR NEUROLOGICAL HEALTH 91

CHAPTER 17
PROTECTING AND HEALING THE NERVOUS SYSTEM 93
DMSO for Nerve Regeneration and Repair 93
Treating Carpal Tunnel, Sciatica, and Chronic Headaches 94

CHAPTER 18
DMSO AND COGNITIVE FUNCTION 97
Investigating DMSO for Alzheimer's and Dementia Prevention 97
Enhancing Brain Circulation and Reducing Neuroinflammation 99

BOOK 10
DMSO FOR DETOX AND HEAVY METAL REMOVAL 101

CHAPTER 19
DMSO AS A DETOXIFYING AGENT 103
How DMSO Binds to and Eliminates Heavy Metals 103
Supporting Liver and Kidney Function During Detox 104

CHAPTER 20
ADVANCED DETOX PROTOCOLS WITH DMSO 107
Combining DMSO with Activated Charcoal and Vitamin C 107
Safely Implementing a Long-Term Detox Plan 108

BOOK 11
DMSO IN CANCER THERAPY SUPPORT 111

CHAPTER 21
HOW DMSO ASSISTS CANCER TREATMENT 113
Enhancing Chemotherapy Absorption While Reducing Side Effects 113
DMSO and Oxygen Therapy: Improving Cellular Oxygenation 114

CHAPTER 22
ALTERNATIVE CANCER PROTOCOLS WITH DMSO 117
Combining DMSO with High-Dose Vitamin C and Herbal Treatments 117
Success Stories of DMSO in Cancer Support 118

BOOK 12
DMSO FOR VETERINARY USE 121

CHAPTER 23
TREATING PETS AND LIVESTOCK WITH DMSO 123
Arthritis, Inflammation, and Injury Recovery in Animals 123
Safe Dosages for Dogs, Cats, and Horses 124

CHAPTER 24
ADVANCED VETERINARY APPLICATIONS 127
DMSO for Equine Performance and Racehorse Recovery 127
Treating Skin Conditions and Infections in Pets 128

BOOK 13
HIGH-DOSE DMSO THERAPY AND CLINICAL APPLICATIONS 131

CHAPTER 25
ADVANCED CLINICAL USES OF DMSO 133
DMSO Therapy for Lyme Disease and Chronic Conditions 133
Case Studies on High-Dose Treatment Safety 134

CHAPTER 26
COMBINING DMSO WITH OTHER ADVANCED THERAPIES 137
Synergistic Effects with Ozone, Hydrogen Peroxide, and Chelation Therapy 137
Emerging Research on Future Applications 138

BOOK 14
THE CONTROVERSY SURROUNDING DMSO 141

CHAPTER 27
WHY DMSO REMAINS CONTROVERSIAL 143
The Role of the FDA and Pharmaceutical Industry 143
Addressing Common Myths and Misconceptions 144

CHAPTER 28
THE LEGAL AND ETHICAL LANDSCAPE OF DMSO 147
Regulations in the U.S. and Worldwide 147
Ensuring Safe and Responsible Use 149

BOOK 15
DMSO REMEDIES FOR EYE HEALTH (CATARACTS, VISION RESTORATION) 153

CHAPTER 29
TARGETED DMSO APPLICATIONS FOR VISION SUPPORT 155
DMSO Eye Compress for Cataract Clarity 155
Aloe Vera & DMSO Blend for Dry Eyes Relief 156
Castor Oil & DMSO Solution for Retinal Support 156
Herbal DMSO Rinse for Eye Fatigue and Strain 156
Vitamin C & DMSO Eye Pad for Oxidative Stress Reduction 157
MSM & DMSO Eye Drop Alternative for Lubrication 157
Bilberry Extract & DMSO Topical Application for Vision Enhancement 157
Chamomile & DMSO Cold Compress for Reducing Eye Inflammation 158
DMSO & Saline Wash for Gentle Eye Detoxification 158
Coconut Water & DMSO Eye Soothing Formula 158

BOOK 16
DMSO REMEDIES FOR DIGESTIVE DISORDERS (IBS, CROHN'S DISEASE) 159

CHAPTER 30
DMSO PROTOCOLS FOR GUT HEALTH AND DIGESTIVE RECOVERY 161
DMSO & Aloe Vera Drink for Gut Lining Support 161
Chamomile & DMSO Infusion for IBS Symptom Relief 162
Slippery Elm & DMSO Blend for Soothing Intestinal Inflammation 162
Coconut Water & DMSO Hydration Therapy for Digestive Balance 162
DMSO & Marshmallow Root Formula for Ulcer Protection 163
Peppermint Oil & DMSO Stomach Massage for Bloating Reduction 163
Probiotic Yogurt & DMSO Topical Application for Gut Microbiome Support 163
Ginger & DMSO Compress for Reducing Abdominal Discomfort 164
Bone Broth & DMSO Elixir for Intestinal Healing 164
Licorice Root & DMSO Solution for Acid Reflux Control 164

BOOK 17
DMSO REMEDIES FOR RESPIRATORY HEALTH (ASTHMA, COPD) 165

CHAPTER 31
STRENGTHENING LUNG FUNCTION WITH DMSO THERAPIES 167
DMSO & Eucalyptus Steam Inhalation for Clearer Airways 167
Honey & DMSO Chest Rub for Respiratory Comfort 168
Peppermint & DMSO Vapor Rub for Sinus and Lung Relief 168
Saline & DMSO Nebulizer Solution for Lung Hydration 168
Turmeric & DMSO Gargle for Throat and Bronchial Support 169
Magnesium Oil & DMSO Topical Blend for Respiratory Muscle Relaxation 169
Ginger & DMSO Warm Compress for Chest Congestion 169
Licorice Root & DMSO Tonic for Lung Inflammation Control 170
Aloe Vera & DMSO Drink for Mucosal Lining Protection 170
Thyme & DMSO Herbal Infusion for Bronchial Support 170

BOOK 18
DMSO REMEDIES FOR SURGERY AND RECOVERY (PREVENTING POST-OP INFECTIONS) 171

CHAPTER 32
POST-SURGICAL HEALING AND INFECTION PREVENTION WITH DMSO 173
DMSO & Aloe Vera Gel for Scar Reduction and Skin Regeneration 173
Honey & DMSO Wound Dressing for Natural Antibacterial Protection 174
Chamomile & DMSO Compress for Post-Surgical Swelling Control 174
Coconut Oil & DMSO Blend for Skin Hydration and Healing Support 174

Collagen & DMSO Topical Solution for Tissue Repair Enhancement 175
Turmeric & DMSO Infused Oil for Reducing Post-Op Inflammation 175
Saline & DMSO Spray for Gentle Wound Cleansing 175
MSM & DMSO Lotion for Pain Relief and Recovery Acceleration 176
Green Tea Extract & DMSO Serum for Skin Soothing and Repair 176
Vitamin E & DMSO Scar Treatment for Enhanced Healing 176

BOOK 19
DMSO REMEDIES FOR SYNERGY WITH OXYGEN, MSM, AND NATURAL THERAPIES 177

CHAPTER 33
ENHANCING DMSO'S EFFECTS WITH NATURAL HEALING COMBINATIONS 179
DMSO & MSM Lotion for Joint Flexibility and Pain Relief 179
Hydrogen Peroxide & DMSO Solution for Skin and Wound Oxygenation 180
Ozone-Infused Olive Oil & DMSO Blend for Antimicrobial Support 180
Magnesium & DMSO Spray for Muscle Relaxation and Recovery 180
Coenzyme Q10 & DMSO Topical Application for Cellular Energy Boost 181
Chlorella & DMSO Detox Formula for Heavy Metal Removal 181
Arnica & DMSO Gel for Bruise and Inflammation Recovery 181
Omega-3 & DMSO Massage Oil for Cardiovascular and Anti-Inflammatory Benefits 182
Vitamin C & DMSO Serum for Skin Regeneration and Antioxidant Protection 182
Ashwagandha & DMSO Adaptogenic Blend for Stress and Immune Support 182

BOOK 20
FINAL THOUGHTS AND PERSONALIZED HEALING PLANS 183

CHAPTER 34
CUSTOMIZING DMSO TREATMENTS FOR INDIVIDUAL NEEDS 185
How to Create Your Own Protocols 185
Adjusting Dosages Based on Health Conditions 187

CHAPTER 35
THE FUTURE OF DMSO IN NATURAL MEDICINE 191
Emerging Research and New Applications 191
How to Safely Integrate DMSO Into a Holistic Health Plan 192

YOUR EXCLUSIVE BONUS 196

BOOK 1
THE SCIENCE BEHIND DMSO – UNDERSTANDING THE HEALING MOLECULE

CHAPTER 1
WHAT IS DMSO AND HOW DOES IT WORK?

The Unique Chemical Structure and Its Role in Healing

Dimethyl sulfoxide (DMSO) is a remarkable molecule with a unique chemical structure that grants it a wide range of therapeutic properties. Unlike most conventional treatments, DMSO operates at a cellular level, penetrating tissues deeply and interacting directly with biological processes. Understanding its structure helps explain why it is so effective in healing and pain relief.

DMSO's molecular formula is C_2H_6OS, and it consists of three essential components:

- **Two methyl groups (-CH$_3$):** These small, nonpolar groups contribute to DMSO's ability to interact with both water-soluble and fat-soluble compounds.
- **A sulfur-oxygen (S=O) functional group:** This highly polar group gives DMSO its strong affinity for water and biological membranes, allowing it to dissolve both hydrophilic and hydrophobic substances.
- **A sulfur atom (S):** This is the key to DMSO's anti-inflammatory and antioxidant properties, as sulfur plays a crucial role in detoxification and cellular repair.

Molecular Behavior: Why DMSO Acts Differently Than Other Compounds

DMSO exhibits unusual chemical behavior that makes it unlike any other therapeutic agent:

- **Highly Soluble in Water and Lipids:** DMSO can dissolve both water-soluble (hydrophilic) and fat-soluble (lipophilic) substances, allowing it to transport a wide range of therapeutic compounds directly into cells.
- **Rapid Absorption Through the Skin:** Unlike most topical treatments, DMSO passes through the skin almost instantly without damaging cell membranes. This makes it an ideal carrier for delivering other medications or supplements deep into the tissues.
- **Cryoprotective Properties:** DMSO prevents cellular damage from freezing, which is why it is commonly used to preserve human cells, tissues, and even stem cells in medical applications.
- **Powerful Solvent Capabilities:** DMSO can dissolve a vast range of organic and inorganic compounds, making it a highly adaptable compound for medical and industrial use.

How DMSO Interacts with the Body's Biological Systems

DMSO's small molecular size and high polarity allow it to cross biological barriers that most drugs cannot penetrate. This includes:

- **The skin barrier:** DMSO moves through skin layers into the bloodstream within seconds, making it an efficient transdermal delivery system.
- **Cell membranes:** Unlike many therapeutic agents that require transport proteins, DMSO diffuses freely across cell membranes, allowing for rapid intracellular activity.
- **The blood-brain barrier (BBB):** Few substances can pass through the protective shield of the brain, but DMSO easily crosses the BBB, making it a valuable agent for neurological treatments.

The Role of DMSO in Cellular Healing and Inflammation Reduction

DMSO's interaction with cells triggers a cascade of beneficial effects, including:

- **Reducing oxidative stress:** DMSO is a potent free radical scavenger, neutralizing harmful molecules that cause cellular aging and inflammation.
- **Modulating immune response:** It regulates the activity of immune cells, preventing excessive inflammation while still allowing the body to fight infections.
- **Enhancing nutrient absorption:** DMSO improves the uptake of essential vitamins, minerals, and other healing compounds, boosting cellular function and repair.
- **Reducing pain signals:** By inhibiting the transmission of pain-inducing neurotransmitters, DMSO provides rapid relief from chronic pain conditions like arthritis and nerve damage.

Structural Advantage: Why DMSO Works Better Than Other Anti-Inflammatory Agents

PROPERTY	DMSO	NSAIDS (E.G., IBUPROFEN)	STEROIDS
Cellular Penetration	High	Low	Medium
Anti-Inflammatory Action	Strong	Moderate	Strong
Side Effects	Minimal (if used correctly)	Gastrointestinal irritation, kidney stress	Immune suppression, hormonal imbalance
Time to Take Effect	Fast (minutes to hours)	Moderate (hours)	Slow (days)

DMSO stands out because it provides fast-acting relief without the severe side effects associated with long-term steroid or NSAID use. It works directly at the site of inflammation, rather than just masking symptoms.

DMSO's chemical uniqueness is the foundation of its healing capabilities. Its ability to penetrate biological barriers, transport therapeutic compounds, and modulate inflammation makes it a powerful tool in natural medicine.

Why DMSO Is So Effective: A Deep Dive into Its Mechanism

Dimethyl sulfoxide (DMSO) is a highly versatile therapeutic compound known for its rapid penetration, powerful anti-inflammatory properties, and ability to transport other molecules directly into tissues. Unlike conventional pain relievers or anti-inflammatory drugs, DMSO doesn't merely mask symptoms—it actively works at a cellular level to promote healing. This unique effectiveness can be traced to three primary mechanisms: cellular permeability, anti-inflammatory action, and neurological modulation.

Unmatched Cellular Penetration: The Key to Rapid Absorption

One of the most remarkable characteristics of DMSO is its ability to effortlessly pass through biological membranes. This is due to its high polarity and small molecular size, allowing it to:

- **Absorb through the skin in seconds:** Unlike topical creams that take time to diffuse, DMSO enters the bloodstream almost immediately after application.
- **Transport other therapeutic agents:** DMSO can carry vitamins, minerals, and even pharmaceuticals deep into tissues, enhancing their effectiveness.
- **Cross the blood-brain barrier (BBB):** Very few substances can penetrate the protective barrier surrounding the brain. DMSO does this naturally, allowing it to deliver neurological benefits that most drugs cannot achieve.

DMSO's ability to directly reach affected areas makes it far more effective than oral or injected medications, which must first pass through the digestive system or bloodstream before reaching target tissues. This direct, localized action is why many individuals experience relief within minutes of application.

Anti-Inflammatory Action: How DMSO Stops the Root Cause of Pain

Inflammation is the underlying factor in many chronic conditions, from arthritis to autoimmune disorders. Unlike NSAIDs, which suppress inflammation temporarily, DMSO actively modulates the body's inflammatory response. It does this by:

- **Blocking inflammatory cytokines:** DMSO inhibits interleukin-6 (IL-6) and tumor necrosis factor-alpha (TNF-α), two compounds heavily involved in chronic inflammation.
- **Reducing oxidative stress:** DMSO is a potent free radical scavenger, neutralizing harmful molecules that damage cells and accelerate aging.
- **Improving circulation and oxygen delivery:** By expanding blood vessels and reducing cellular swelling, DMSO enhances oxygen flow to damaged tissues, accelerating recovery.

These effects make DMSO particularly valuable for individuals suffering from joint pain, muscle injuries, and inflammatory diseases where conventional treatments often fall short.

Neurological Modulation: DMSO's Role in Pain Perception and Nerve Repair

Beyond reducing inflammation, DMSO has a direct impact on the nervous system, making it especially useful for neuropathy, sciatica, and post-surgical nerve pain. It achieves this through:

- **Blocking pain signal transmission:** DMSO interferes with C-fiber nerve conduction, preventing the intensity of pain signals from reaching the brain.
- **Regenerating damaged nerve tissue:** Research suggests that DMSO stimulates nerve growth factor (NGF), a protein critical for nerve repair and regeneration.
- **Enhancing cellular hydration:** Nerve cells rely on proper hydration and electrolyte balance. DMSO improves cellular water retention, keeping nerve tissues functional and healthy.

This mechanism explains why DMSO provides pain relief without the side effects of opioids or sedatives. Instead of dulling sensations, it corrects the underlying dysfunction at a cellular level.

Why DMSO Works Faster and More Effectively Than Traditional Treatments

MECHANISM OF ACTION	DMSO	NSAIDS (IBUPROFEN, ASPIRIN)	OPIOIDS (MORPHINE, OXYCODONE)
Cellular penetration	Rapid, crosses membranes instantly	Limited to bloodstream	No cellular penetration
Inflammation control	Blocks cytokines, improves circulation	Blocks enzymes, temporary relief	No anti-inflammatory effect
Pain relief mechanism	Modulates nerve conduction	Blocks pain at the peripheral level	Alters brain chemistry, addictive
Time to take effect	Minutes	Hours	Hours
Side effects	Minimal with proper use	Stomach ulcers, kidney stress	Dependency, sedation

Unlike pharmaceuticals, DMSO does not disrupt normal bodily functions—it works with the body to heal, rather than just managing symptoms. This fundamental difference is what makes it such an effective and natural option for pain relief, inflammation control, and nerve repair.

CHAPTER 2

THE HISTORY AND MEDICAL EVOLUTION OF DMSO

From Industrial Solvent to Medical Marvel: The Journey of DMSO

Dimethyl sulfoxide (DMSO) has one of the most unexpected origins in medical history. Today, it is widely recognized for its anti-inflammatory, analgesic, and healing properties, yet it was not originally discovered for medical use. Instead, DMSO was first identified as a byproduct of the paper industry, and its journey from industrial solvent to medical breakthrough is a story filled with scientific curiosity, groundbreaking discoveries, and regulatory controversies.

The Accidental Discovery of DMSO

DMSO was first synthesized in the mid-19th century by the Russian chemist Alexander Zaytsev. At the time, its potential applications were unknown, and it remained largely a chemical curiosity rather than a subject of serious research.

However, it wasn't until the 20th century that scientists started recognizing DMSO's unique properties. Because of its ability to dissolve both organic and inorganic compounds, it became widely used in the paper, textile, and pharmaceutical industries as a powerful solvent.

Breakthrough in Medical Research: The 1950s and 1960s

The transition of DMSO from an industrial compound to a medical marvel began in the 1950s, when Dr. Stanley Jacob, a surgeon and researcher at the Oregon Health & Science University, became interested in its biological effects. Initially, Dr. Jacob was investigating better ways to preserve organs for transplantation. While experimenting with DMSO, he discovered something unexpected:

- DMSO penetrated the skin almost instantly without damaging it.
- It transported other substances through the skin and into the bloodstream.
- It had remarkable anti-inflammatory and pain-relieving effects.

These findings led Dr. Jacob to explore its therapeutic potential. His research revealed that DMSO reduced swelling, relieved pain, and accelerated wound healing, making it a promising treatment for arthritis, injuries, and nerve-related conditions.

The Explosion of Interest in the 1960s

By the early 1960s, the medical community had become fascinated by DMSO's potential. Researchers began exploring its effects on a range of conditions, from burn treatment to neurological disorders. The results were promising:

- DMSO was shown to protect cells from damage, making it useful in cryopreservation for storing organs and tissues.
- It demonstrated neuroprotective properties, showing potential for spinal cord injuries and stroke recovery.
- It relieved chronic pain and inflammation in conditions like arthritis and fibromyalgia.

The excitement surrounding DMSO was so intense that over 1,000 scientific articles were published within a few years, leading many to believe that it could become a mainstay in modern medicine.

Regulatory Setbacks and Controversy

Despite these promising discoveries, DMSO's rise in medicine was abruptly halted in the mid-1960s. After reports surfaced of temporary eye irritation in animal studies, the FDA placed restrictions on its medical use in the United States. While many scientists—including Dr. Jacob—argued that the benefits far outweighed the risks, regulatory agencies remained skeptical.

Although the medical research on DMSO never stopped, it was overshadowed by pharmaceutical alternatives, and its use became limited primarily to veterinary medicine and alternative health communities.

Yet, despite regulatory hurdles, DMSO's legacy as a powerful healing agent remains undeniable. The same solvent that once powered the paper industry has evolved into one of the most intriguing and misunderstood compounds in medical science.

Why Mainstream Medicine Overlooks DMSO: Regulations and Politics

Despite its remarkable therapeutic properties, DMSO remains largely ignored by mainstream medicine. Unlike many pharmaceutical drugs that quickly gain FDA approval and widespread acceptance, DMSO has faced regulatory barriers, skepticism, and political resistance for decades. Its journey through the medical system reveals a complex web of safety concerns, pharmaceutical industry interests, and bureaucratic obstacles that have kept it from becoming a standard treatment.

The 1960s FDA Controversy and the First Clinical Setback

The turning point in DMSO's medical history came in the 1960s, when early research by Dr. Stanley Jacob and other scientists demonstrated its anti-inflammatory, pain-relieving, and cellular protective effects. These discoveries led to high hopes for FDA approval, and clinical trials were set in motion.

However, in 1965, reports surfaced of temporary eye changes in laboratory animals treated with high doses of DMSO. While these changes were not associated with vision loss or long-term damage, they were enough for the FDA to suspend human trials.

- **No confirmed human toxicity:** Despite extensive studies, no serious adverse effects were found in human subjects.
- **Animal study concerns:** The FDA used uncertain findings in animal research to justify restrictions.
- **Medical community frustration:** Many researchers, including Dr. Jacob, argued that DMSO was far safer than many approved medications at the time.

The FDA's sudden suspension of trials led to a decline in funding for DMSO research, forcing many scientists to abandon their work.

The Role of the Pharmaceutical Industry in Suppressing DMSO

Unlike patented pharmaceutical drugs, DMSO is a naturally occurring substance, meaning it cannot be exclusively patented by any one company. This lack of financial incentive has played a crucial role in its exclusion from mainstream medicine.

- **No monopoly, no profits:** Pharmaceutical companies focus on highly profitable drugs, often at the expense of older, unpatentable treatments.
- **Competition with anti-inflammatory drugs:** NSAIDs, opioids, and corticosteroids generate billions in revenue, while DMSO offers similar or superior benefits without severe side effects.
- **Lack of corporate funding:** Without the backing of major pharmaceutical firms, DMSO research struggles to secure large-scale clinical trials.

The absence of a strong financial motive means that drug companies have little interest in promoting DMSO, despite its proven therapeutic value.

Regulatory Challenges: A Slow and Limited Approval Process

Though DMSO remains widely used in veterinary medicine and as a cryoprotectant in organ preservation, its approval for human medical use has been slow and limited.

YEAR	REGULATORY STATUS	KEY EVENTS
1978	FDA Approves DMSO for Interstitial Cystitis	First and only FDA-approved human treatment
1980s	Global Recognition	Used for various conditions in **Europe, Russia, and South America**
Present	Still Restricted in the U.S.	Allowed for **veterinary use, alternative medicine, and research**

Despite decades of scientific support, the FDA has refused to expand approvals beyond a single bladder condition, while many other countries allow wider medical use.

Why Physicians Avoid Recommending DMSO

Beyond regulations, mainstream physicians rarely recommend DMSO, largely due to:

- **Lack of medical school education:** Most doctors are never taught about DMSO's properties in their training.
- **Fear of legal repercussions:** Since DMSO is not widely approved, doctors risk scrutiny for recommending it.
- **Influence of pharmaceutical-sponsored research:** Medical guidelines are shaped by drug-funded studies, which often exclude unpatentable substances like DMSO.

The medical system's reliance on pharmaceutical-driven research and FDA approval processes has kept DMSO on the fringes of mainstream treatment, despite its extraordinary potential.

BOOK 2
DMSO FOR CHRONIC PAIN RELIEF

CHAPTER 3
THE ROLE OF DMSO IN PAIN MANAGEMENT

How DMSO Blocks Pain Signals and Reduces Inflammation

DMSO's ability to relieve pain and inflammation is one of its most powerful and widely studied effects. Unlike traditional painkillers that temporarily suppress symptoms, DMSO works at the cellular level, directly targeting the root causes of pain and inflammation. This dual-action mechanism sets it apart from pharmaceuticals, making it a natural yet highly effective alternative for managing both acute and chronic pain conditions.

How DMSO Interrupts Pain Transmission

Pain is the result of signals traveling through the nervous system, alerting the brain to tissue damage or dysfunction. These signals are carried by nerve fibers, particularly C-fibers and A-delta fibers, which transmit pain sensations from the affected area to the brain.

DMSO blocks pain at its source, rather than simply numbing the affected area. It achieves this by:

- **Inhibiting pain signal transmission:** DMSO disrupts the conduction of pain impulses along nerve fibers, preventing them from reaching the brain. This mechanism is particularly useful for conditions involving nerve pain (neuropathy), arthritis, and muscle injuries.
- **Blocking inflammatory chemicals:** When tissue is damaged, the body releases substances like bradykinin, histamine, and prostaglandins, which increase pain sensitivity. DMSO neutralizes these compounds, reducing pain perception.
- **Modulating sodium channels in nerves:** Pain signals rely on sodium ions to transmit electrical impulses. DMSO alters sodium channel function, effectively reducing the ability of nerves to send pain messages.

This rapid interruption of pain transmission makes DMSO one of the fastest-acting natural pain relievers available, often providing relief within minutes of application.

DMSO's Anti-Inflammatory Power: Stopping Pain at Its Source

Inflammation is the body's natural response to injury, infection, or chronic conditions. However, excessive or persistent inflammation leads to pain, swelling, and tissue damage. DMSO's effectiveness in reducing inflammation is due to its ability to:

- **Inhibit inflammatory cytokines:** DMSO suppresses tumor necrosis factor-alpha (TNF-α), interleukin-6 (IL-6), and prostaglandins, which are key players in chronic inflammation.
- **Reduce oxidative stress:** Inflammation generates free radicals, which damage cells and prolong pain. DMSO acts as a potent antioxidant, neutralizing these harmful molecules.
- **Improve blood circulation:** By dilating blood vessels and increasing oxygen supply to tissues, DMSO helps flush out inflammatory byproducts, accelerating healing.

Unlike NSAIDs, which primarily block COX enzymes, DMSO works through multiple pathways, addressing both the cause of inflammation and its painful symptoms.

Why DMSO Works Where Other Pain Relievers Fail

Many conventional painkillers only mask symptoms, requiring repeated doses that can cause dependency or long-term health risks. DMSO, on the other hand:

- Targets both nerve conduction and inflammation, providing more comprehensive pain relief.
- Works transdermally, meaning it can be applied directly to the affected area without affecting other organs.
- Does not cause gastrointestinal issues, unlike NSAIDs, which can lead to ulcers and stomach irritation.

By directly addressing the underlying mechanisms of pain, DMSO stands out as a safe, effective, and scientifically backed alternative for those seeking long-term relief without harmful side effects.

Comparing DMSO to NSAIDs and Opioids: The Safer Alternative

Chronic pain affects millions of people worldwide, and for decades, mainstream medicine has relied on NSAIDs (nonsteroidal anti-inflammatory drugs) and opioids to manage discomfort. While these drugs can offer relief, they also come with significant side effects, long-term health risks, and even dependency issues. DMSO, on the other hand, provides a natural, effective, and safer alternative that works at the cellular level to address pain without the dangers associated with conventional treatments.

How NSAIDs Work and Their Limitations

NSAIDs, such as ibuprofen, naproxen, and aspirin, are among the most commonly used pain relievers. They work by inhibiting cyclooxygenase (COX) enzymes, which are responsible for producing prostaglandins—compounds that trigger inflammation and pain.

While NSAIDs can be effective for short-term relief of mild to moderate pain, their long-term use poses significant risks, including:

- **Gastrointestinal damage:** NSAIDs can irritate the stomach lining, leading to ulcers, acid reflux, and even gastrointestinal bleeding.

- **Kidney stress:** Prolonged use of NSAIDs has been linked to reduced kidney function and an increased risk of kidney disease.
- **Cardiovascular complications:** Some NSAIDs, particularly selective COX-2 inhibitors, have been shown to increase the risk of heart attacks and strokes.

DMSO differs significantly because it does not inhibit COX enzymes, meaning it does not interfere with the body's natural healing processes. Instead, it reduces inflammation at the source while also improving cellular oxygenation and circulation, accelerating tissue repair.

Opioids: A Dangerous Path to Pain Relief

Opioids such as oxycodone, morphine, and fentanyl are commonly prescribed for severe or chronic pain. Unlike NSAIDs, which reduce inflammation, opioids work by binding to opioid receptors in the brain and spinal cord, blocking the sensation of pain.

Although opioids can be effective for short-term acute pain, they come with severe drawbacks, including:

- **High risk of addiction:** Opioids alter brain chemistry, leading to dependency and withdrawal symptoms. Many patients find themselves unable to stop using them even when their original pain subsides.
- **Tolerance and escalating doses:** Over time, patients require higher doses to achieve the same level of pain relief, increasing the risk of overdose.
- **Respiratory depression:** One of the most dangerous effects of opioids is their ability to slow breathing, which can be fatal in cases of overdose.

Unlike opioids, DMSO does not alter brain chemistry or create dependency. It works directly at the site of pain and inflammation, addressing the root cause rather than masking symptoms.

Why DMSO Is the Safer and More Effective Option

DMSO stands apart from NSAIDs and opioids because it naturally relieves pain while promoting healing. Unlike NSAIDs, it does not damage the stomach or kidneys, and unlike opioids, it does not carry the risk of addiction or overdose.

By reducing inflammation, improving circulation, and blocking pain signals at the cellular level, DMSO presents a powerful, science-backed alternative to traditional painkillers—without the dangerous side effects.

CHAPTER 4
USING DMSO FOR ARTHRITIS, FIBROMYALGIA, AND NEUROPATHY

Targeting Joint Pain and Stiffness with DMSO Protocols

Chronic joint pain and stiffness are among the most debilitating symptoms for individuals suffering from conditions like arthritis, osteoarthritis, and fibromyalgia. These conditions limit mobility, impact quality of life, and often require long-term pain management strategies. Conventional treatments such as NSAIDs, corticosteroids, and physical therapy may offer temporary relief but often come with side effects and diminishing effectiveness over time.

DMSO provides a natural, science-backed alternative that not only reduces pain but also targets inflammation and supports tissue repair. Its ability to penetrate deep into joints, modulate inflammatory responses, and improve circulation makes it an ideal therapeutic option for those seeking long-term relief.

How DMSO Addresses Joint Pain and Stiffness

Joint pain and stiffness are driven by inflammation, cartilage breakdown, and reduced synovial fluid production. DMSO works through multiple mechanisms to counteract these underlying issues:

- **Reduces inflammatory cytokines:** DMSO inhibits pro-inflammatory molecules such as interleukin-6 (IL-6) and tumor necrosis factor-alpha (TNF-α), which contribute to swelling and pain.
- **Improves synovial fluid function:** The lubricating fluid within joints is essential for smooth movement. DMSO penetrates joint capsules, enhancing fluid mobility and reducing stiffness.
- **Alleviates oxidative stress:** Free radicals contribute to joint degradation and cartilage breakdown. DMSO acts as an antioxidant, neutralizing oxidative damage and slowing joint deterioration.
- **Enhances blood circulation:** By improving microvascular flow, DMSO helps deliver oxygen and nutrients to damaged joints, accelerating healing.

Unlike oral medications, which must pass through the digestive system and may take hours to act, DMSO works within minutes, making it an ideal solution for immediate relief from joint discomfort.

Why DMSO Is Ideal for Arthritis and Osteoarthritis

Arthritis, particularly osteoarthritis and rheumatoid arthritis, is characterized by chronic joint inflammation, cartilage erosion, and progressive pain. Traditional treatment options often fail to halt the degenerative process, leaving patients dependent on medication for symptom control.

DMSO, however, provides three key advantages for arthritis sufferers:

- **Slows cartilage degradation:** By reducing inflammation and oxidative stress, DMSO helps preserve cartilage health and may slow the progression of arthritis.
- **Acts as a natural analgesic:** Unlike opioids or NSAIDs, which mask pain, DMSO works at the cellular level to block pain signals without causing dependency.
- **Provides long-lasting relief:** Regular use of DMSO has been associated with reduced flare-ups, improved joint flexibility, and sustained mobility benefits.

This makes DMSO a powerful tool for those seeking both immediate pain relief and long-term joint health improvements.

DMSO for Fibromyalgia-Related Joint Discomfort

Fibromyalgia is a complex pain condition that affects muscles, joints, and connective tissues. Unlike arthritis, which is primarily inflammatory, fibromyalgia involves centralized pain processing dysfunction. However, many fibromyalgia patients experience joint stiffness, swelling, and limited mobility, making DMSO a viable treatment option.

For fibromyalgia sufferers, DMSO works by:

- **Reducing neurogenic inflammation:** DMSO helps dampen nerve hypersensitivity, which is a major contributor to fibromyalgia pain.
- **Improving mitochondrial function:** Cellular energy dysfunction is common in fibromyalgia, and DMSO helps restore normal cellular metabolism, reducing fatigue and stiffness.
- **Providing targeted relief without systemic side effects:** Many fibromyalgia medications cause brain fog, drowsiness, or dizziness, while DMSO delivers pain relief without cognitive impairment.

Its ability to address both inflammatory and neuropathic pain makes DMSO one of the most comprehensive natural therapies for fibromyalgia-related joint and muscle discomfort.

By incorporating DMSO into joint pain management protocols, individuals with arthritis, osteoarthritis, and fibromyalgia can experience greater mobility, less pain, and a better quality of life—without the long-term risks associated with pharmaceutical treatments.

Healing Nerve Damage: DMSO for Neuropathy and Sciatica

Nerve damage is one of the most difficult and frustrating conditions to manage, often resulting in chronic pain, numbness, burning sensations, and reduced mobility. Neuropathy, whether caused by diabetes, autoimmune disorders, or injury, can severely impact daily life. Sciatica, on the other hand, is a condition involving compression or irritation of the sciatic nerve, leading to radiating pain, weakness, and discomfort that extends from the lower back down the leg.

Traditional treatments for nerve pain often rely on prescription drugs like gabapentin, opioids, or corticosteroids, which may temporarily mask symptoms but fail to heal nerve damage. DMSO offers a unique and natural solution, not only by reducing pain and inflammation but also by supporting nerve regeneration and restoring function at a cellular level.

How DMSO Supports Nerve Healing

Unlike many conventional treatments that simply block nerve signals, DMSO works at the root of nerve dysfunction. It enhances the body's natural healing mechanisms by:

- **Reducing nerve inflammation:** Chronic nerve pain is often caused by swelling and pressure around damaged nerves. DMSO penetrates deeply into tissues, reducing inflammation in the affected area and alleviating nerve compression.
- **Enhancing cellular repair:** Nerves rely on efficient nutrient delivery and oxygenation to regenerate. DMSO improves blood flow and oxygen uptake, creating an optimal environment for damaged nerve cells to repair and rebuild.
- **Modulating pain signals:** Unlike opioids, which work at the central nervous system level, DMSO directly blocks the transmission of pain signals from damaged nerves. It calms overactive nerve activity, reducing burning sensations, tingling, and sharp pain.
- **Protecting against oxidative stress:** Neuropathy is often worsened by free radical damage, which further deteriorates nerve function. DMSO acts as a potent antioxidant, neutralizing harmful molecules that contribute to nerve degeneration.

These combined effects make DMSO one of the most promising options for nerve pain management, particularly for peripheral neuropathy, sciatica, and nerve compression syndromes.

DMSO for Peripheral Neuropathy

Peripheral neuropathy affects the nerves outside of the brain and spinal cord, commonly causing tingling, numbness, and loss of sensation. This condition is particularly common in diabetics and those suffering from autoimmune diseases or chemotherapy-induced nerve damage.

DMSO's effectiveness in treating peripheral neuropathy stems from its ability to:

- Reduce nerve swelling, alleviating pressure on affected nerve endings.
- Improve nerve conductivity, allowing damaged nerves to send and receive signals more efficiently.
- Restore sensation, particularly in cases where neuropathy has led to numbness or hypersensitivity.

Regular application of DMSO has been reported to significantly improve nerve function, allowing individuals to regain movement and sensation in affected areas.

DMSO for Sciatica and Compressed Nerve Pain

Sciatica occurs when the sciatic nerve—the longest nerve in the body—is compressed or irritated, usually due to a herniated disc, spinal misalignment, or muscle tension. The pain often radiates from the lower back down the leg, creating intense discomfort and limited mobility.

DMSO can help alleviate sciatic nerve pain by:

- Reducing inflammation around the spinal discs, which can ease nerve compression.
- Relaxing tight muscles, preventing further irritation of the sciatic nerve.
- Encouraging nerve healing, preventing long-term damage from chronic compression.

By targeting inflammation, promoting nerve repair, and improving circulation, DMSO provides a safer, long-term alternative for individuals seeking relief from neuropathic pain and sciatica without relying on pharmaceuticals.

BOOK 3
DMSO FOR INJURY RECOVERY AND POST-SURGICAL HEALING

CHAPTER 5
SPEEDING UP HEALING WITH DMSO

How DMSO Reduces Swelling and Bruising Post-Injury

Swelling and bruising are natural responses to injury, but they often prolong pain and delay healing. After a trauma—whether from a fall, muscle strain, or joint sprain—the body triggers an inflammatory response to protect the affected area. Blood vessels expand, immune cells rush in, and fluid accumulates, causing swelling, discoloration, and stiffness. While inflammation is part of the healing process, excessive or prolonged swelling can lead to increased pain, reduced mobility, and a slower recovery.

DMSO is unique in its ability to penetrate deep into tissues, reduce inflammation, and enhance circulation, making it a powerful tool for minimizing post-injury swelling and bruising. Unlike traditional anti-inflammatory medications that act systemically, DMSO works locally and efficiently, directly targeting the injured area.

The Science Behind DMSO's Anti-Inflammatory Action

One of the key ways DMSO reduces swelling is by modulating the inflammatory response. When an injury occurs, the body releases pro-inflammatory cytokines like tumor necrosis factor-alpha (TNF-α) and interleukin-6 (IL-6), which increase blood flow and fluid retention around damaged tissues. While this response is essential for healing, excessive inflammation can cause unnecessary pain and prolonged recovery time.

DMSO combats this by:

- **Inhibiting inflammatory mediators:** It blocks the release of cytokines that drive excessive swelling. This helps keep inflammation at a manageable level, allowing for healing without unnecessary discomfort.
- **Reducing capillary leakage:** Bruising occurs when tiny blood vessels (capillaries) break, allowing blood to pool under the skin. DMSO strengthens capillary walls, preventing excessive leakage and reducing the severity of bruising.
- **Enhancing fluid drainage:** By improving lymphatic circulation, DMSO helps flush out excess fluid and cellular waste, preventing swelling from persisting longer than necessary.

Unlike NSAIDs or corticosteroids, which suppress inflammation indiscriminately, DMSO modulates the process, ensuring the body still heals efficiently while avoiding excessive tissue damage.

DMSO's Role in Accelerating Bruise Healing

Bruises form when blood vessels rupture, leading to visible discoloration and tenderness. As the body reabsorbs this leaked blood, bruises fade from dark purple to yellow before disappearing completely. However, this process can take several days or even weeks, depending on the severity of the injury and circulatory health.

DMSO speeds up bruise recovery by:

- Improving microcirculation, ensuring oxygen and nutrients reach damaged tissues faster.
- Breaking down accumulated blood, allowing the body to reabsorb pooled blood more quickly.
- Preventing excessive clotting, reducing the formation of hard, painful knots under the skin.

Many conventional treatments for bruises, such as cold packs and topical creams, provide temporary relief but do not address the underlying mechanisms of healing. DMSO, however, works deep within the tissues, ensuring that bruises heal from the inside out, leading to faster recovery and reduced discomfort.

By reducing inflammation, improving circulation, and accelerating the healing process, DMSO offers a safe, effective alternative to traditional treatments for swelling and bruising after injury.

Enhancing Tissue Repair: DMSO for Sprains, Strains, and Tears

Soft tissue injuries such as sprains, strains, and ligament tears are among the most common musculoskeletal issues, affecting people of all ages and activity levels. These injuries occur when muscles, tendons, or ligaments are overstretched or torn, leading to pain, swelling, and limited mobility. Traditional treatment approaches—such as rest, ice, compression, and elevation (RICE)—may help manage symptoms, but they often fail to accelerate true healing at the cellular level.

DMSO presents a unique and highly effective solution for tissue repair. Unlike painkillers or anti-inflammatory drugs that only mask symptoms, DMSO actively supports the body's natural healing processes, promoting faster recovery, reducing inflammation, and strengthening damaged tissue.

How DMSO Supports Tissue Regeneration

Tissue repair is a complex biological process that involves reducing inflammation, clearing cellular debris, and stimulating new cell growth. DMSO enhances this process by:

- **Increasing cellular permeability:** One of DMSO's defining properties is its ability to penetrate deep into tissues without harming cell membranes. This allows it to deliver oxygen and essential nutrients directly to the site of injury, speeding up the regeneration of damaged fibers.
- **Stimulating collagen production:** Collagen is the primary structural protein responsible for tissue strength and flexibility. DMSO promotes fibroblast activity, leading to stronger, more resilient tissue repair.
- **Reducing fibrotic scarring:** Inadequate healing can result in excessive scar tissue, which weak-

ens injured areas and increases the risk of re-injury. DMSO helps regulate scar tissue formation, ensuring smooth, functional recovery.

By optimizing the body's own repair mechanisms, DMSO accelerates the healing timeline for sprains, strains, and ligament tears while ensuring tissues regain their original strength and elasticity.

DMSO's Role in Pain and Swelling Reduction

Beyond tissue regeneration, pain management and inflammation control are crucial for recovery. Many individuals with soft tissue injuries rely on NSAIDs or corticosteroids, which can have negative long-term effects on joint and muscle health.

DMSO provides effective pain relief by:

- Blocking nerve signal transmission, reducing the intensity of pain.
- Preventing excessive swelling, which can restrict blood flow and slow recovery.
- Neutralizing free radicals, reducing oxidative stress that contributes to prolonged soreness and stiffness.

This multi-faceted approach allows for faster recovery without the side effects of pharmaceuticals, making DMSO a superior option for those looking to heal efficiently.

Why DMSO is Ideal for Athletes and Active Individuals

For individuals who lead active lifestyles, sprains and strains can be a major setback. Athletes, fitness enthusiasts, and even individuals with physically demanding jobs often seek natural yet powerful solutions to return to peak performance as quickly as possible.

DMSO's ability to rapidly reduce swelling, enhance circulation, and restore tissue integrity makes it particularly beneficial for those who cannot afford prolonged downtime. By incorporating DMSO into recovery protocols, individuals can experience less pain, improved mobility, and stronger tissue resilience, reducing the likelihood of chronic injuries or long-term complications.

CHAPTER 6
POST-SURGICAL RECOVERY AND SCAR REDUCTION

Reducing Adhesions and Scar Formation with DMSO

Surgical procedures, whether minor or major, often leave behind scars and adhesions, which can create discomfort, limit mobility, and, in some cases, cause chronic pain. While scarring is a natural part of the body's healing process, excessive or improperly healed scar tissue can lead to tight, raised, or fibrous tissue formations that restrict normal function. Adhesions, on the other hand, occur internally, when scar tissue forms between organs or tissues that should remain separate, often leading to post-surgical complications such as pain and reduced flexibility.

DMSO provides a powerful and natural approach to minimizing the formation of both external scars and internal adhesions. Unlike conventional treatments, which primarily focus on cosmetic scar reduction, DMSO works at a deep tissue level, promoting better collagen formation, reducing fibrosis, and preventing excessive tissue buildup.

How DMSO Prevents Excessive Scar Tissue Formation

Scars form when the body rebuilds damaged tissue by producing collagen, the primary structural protein responsible for wound healing. While collagen is essential for proper recovery, an imbalance in its production can result in raised, rigid, or thick scars that are both unsightly and functionally restrictive.

DMSO helps regulate scar formation through several key mechanisms:

- **Enhancing collagen organization:** Instead of haphazard collagen deposition, DMSO helps align collagen fibers in a structured, flexible manner, preventing hypertrophic and keloid scars.
- **Breaking down excess fibrotic tissue:** When the body produces too much scar tissue, DMSO works to soften and dissolve hardened areas, restoring normal tissue elasticity.
- **Promoting blood circulation:** Proper oxygen and nutrient delivery to healing tissues ensures a smoother, healthier healing process, reducing the risk of thickened scars.

Unlike topical scar creams that only address surface-level healing, DMSO penetrates deep into the tissue layers, ensuring that the entire healing process is regulated from within.

DMSO's Role in Preventing Internal Adhesions

Internal adhesions can develop after surgeries involving the abdomen, pelvis, or joints, where tissue healing leads to fibrous bands forming between organs or muscle layers. These adhesions can cause:

- Chronic pain due to restricted movement of tissues.
- Reduced mobility in joints or muscles affected by excess scar formation.
- Digestive or reproductive issues in cases of abdominal or pelvic adhesions.

DMSO helps prevent and break down adhesions by:

- Softening fibrotic tissue, ensuring that healing tissues do not bond improperly.
- Reducing inflammation at the surgical site, minimizing the triggers for excessive scar tissue development.
- Enhancing cellular hydration, keeping tissues supple and pliable, which discourages adhesion formation.

Patients recovering from joint surgery, C-sections, or abdominal procedures can particularly benefit from DMSO's ability to prevent adhesions and encourage smooth, unrestricted healing.

By regulating the body's healing process at a structural and biochemical level, DMSO ensures that scar tissue remains functional, pliable, and minimal, reducing long-term post-surgical complications.

How DMSO Aids in Post-Surgical Inflammation Control

Surgery, whether minor or major, is a controlled trauma to the body. While necessary for healing and recovery, the post-surgical inflammatory response can often be excessive, painful, and prolonged, leading to swelling, stiffness, and delayed healing. Inflammation is the body's natural defense mechanism, but when left unchecked, it can result in complications such as excessive scar formation, adhesions, and chronic pain.

DMSO offers a unique and effective solution for managing post-surgical inflammation. Unlike traditional anti-inflammatory drugs that suppress the immune response indiscriminately, DMSO works by modulating inflammation, ensuring that the body heals efficiently and without excessive swelling or discomfort.

Understanding Post-Surgical Inflammation and Why It Needs Control

After surgery, the body releases inflammatory cytokines to trigger the healing process. These compounds, including interleukin-6 (IL-6), tumor necrosis factor-alpha (TNF-α), and prostaglandins, promote blood flow, immune cell activation, and tissue regeneration. However, when inflammation becomes excessive, it can:

- Prolong pain and sensitivity, making recovery more difficult.
- Cause fluid buildup, leading to uncomfortable post-surgical swelling.

- Delay tissue regeneration, slowing down the recovery timeline.
- Increase the risk of adhesions, where excess scar tissue forms abnormally between tissues.

Traditional anti-inflammatory drugs, such as NSAIDs or corticosteroids, are often prescribed post-surgery, but they come with side effects like gastrointestinal irritation, kidney stress, and immune suppression. DMSO, in contrast, provides targeted inflammation control without harming the body's natural healing response.

DMSO's Multi-Faceted Approach to Reducing Inflammation

DMSO is a potent anti-inflammatory agent, but unlike conventional medications, it works at multiple levels:

- **Neutralizing inflammatory cytokines:** DMSO reduces the release of TNF-α, IL-6, and other inflammatory mediators, ensuring inflammation remains at a productive rather than destructive level.
- **Improving microcirculation:** DMSO enhances blood flow and oxygen delivery to post-surgical tissues, preventing stagnation and excessive swelling.
- **Acting as a free radical scavenger:** Surgery often leads to oxidative stress, which contributes to prolonged inflammation. DMSO helps neutralize these harmful molecules, allowing for a cleaner, more efficient healing process.

By targeting the root causes of excessive inflammation, DMSO helps patients experience less pain, reduced swelling, and a smoother recovery.

Preventing Complications Associated with Post-Surgical Inflammation

Excessive inflammation doesn't just prolong recovery—it can lead to long-term complications such as chronic pain, fibrosis, and stiffness. DMSO prevents these issues by:

- Keeping tissues hydrated and pliable, reducing the likelihood of excessive scar formation.
- Preventing nerve hypersensitivity, ensuring pain levels remain manageable as the body heals.
- Reducing post-operative stiffness, allowing for greater mobility and faster rehabilitation.

Its ability to penetrate deep into tissues and regulate inflammation at a cellular level makes DMSO one of the most powerful and natural post-surgical recovery tools available, ensuring patients heal faster, with less pain and fewer complications.

BOOK 4
THE ANTI-INFLAMMATORY POWER OF DMSO

CHAPTER 7
INFLAMMATION – THE ROOT OF CHRONIC DISEASE

Understanding Chronic Inflammation and Autoimmune Responses

Inflammation is the body's natural defense mechanism, a necessary process that helps repair tissue, fight infections, and remove harmful invaders. However, when inflammation becomes chronic, it transforms from a protective response into a destructive force, leading to persistent pain, tissue damage, and an increased risk of chronic disease. Many modern health conditions—such as arthritis, fibromyalgia, multiple sclerosis, and inflammatory bowel disease—are driven by ongoing, uncontrolled inflammation that disrupts normal bodily functions.

In some cases, the immune system mistakenly targets the body's own cells, leading to autoimmune diseases where the body's defense mechanisms become a source of harm instead of healing. Understanding the connection between chronic inflammation and autoimmune responses is essential for addressing the root cause of many health conditions rather than just managing symptoms.

How Acute Inflammation Becomes Chronic

Inflammation begins as an essential survival mechanism. When the body detects injury, infection, or toxins, the immune system releases pro-inflammatory molecules, such as cytokines and prostaglandins, to trigger the healing process. This leads to increased blood flow, swelling, redness, and pain, which help protect the affected area while immune cells work to repair the damage.

However, when the initial cause of inflammation is not resolved, or when the body remains in a state of constant immune activation, the inflammatory response fails to shut down properly. Instead of healing tissues, chronic inflammation leads to ongoing tissue destruction and dysfunction. Factors that contribute to persistent inflammation include:

- Unresolved infections that keep the immune system activated.
- Chronic stress, which disrupts immune function and increases inflammatory markers.
- Environmental toxins, such as heavy metals, pesticides, and air pollutants.
- A diet high in processed foods, sugars, and inflammatory fats.
- Gut health imbalances, including leaky gut syndrome and microbiome disruptions.

Over time, chronic inflammation wears down the body's resilience, increasing the risk of conditions such as heart disease, neurodegenerative disorders, autoimmune diseases, and chronic pain syndromes.

The Autoimmune Connection: When the Body Attacks Itself

Autoimmune diseases occur when the immune system mistakenly identifies healthy tissues as threats, launching an immune attack against its own cells. This self-destructive cycle leads to systemic inflammation, tissue damage, and progressive dysfunction in affected organs.

Common autoimmune diseases include:

- **Rheumatoid arthritis (RA):** The immune system attacks joint tissues, leading to inflammation, pain, and progressive joint degeneration.
- **Multiple sclerosis (MS):** The immune system targets the protective myelin sheath around nerves, impairing nervous system function.
- **Hashimoto's thyroiditis:** The immune system attacks the thyroid gland, leading to hormonal imbalances and metabolic dysfunction.
- **Lupus (SLE):** A systemic condition where multiple organs experience inflammation and immune system attacks.

In autoimmune disorders, chronic inflammation is both a cause and a consequence, creating a self-perpetuating cycle where inflammation triggers further immune dysfunction. Breaking this cycle requires regulating inflammation at its source, rather than simply suppressing symptoms with pharmaceutical interventions.

By understanding how chronic inflammation fuels disease and how autoimmune conditions emerge, it becomes clear that the key to true healing lies in restoring balance to the immune system and addressing inflammation at its root cause.

How DMSO Neutralizes Inflammatory Cytokines and Free Radicals

Chronic inflammation is at the core of many debilitating diseases, from autoimmune disorders and arthritis to cardiovascular disease and neurodegenerative conditions. One of the main drivers of inflammation is the overproduction of inflammatory cytokines and free radicals, which damage tissues, accelerate aging, and disrupt immune function. Unlike pharmaceutical anti-inflammatories, which often come with side effects and long-term risks, DMSO works as a powerful natural modulator, reducing inflammation at the source while simultaneously protecting cells from oxidative stress.

DMSO's ability to neutralize harmful inflammatory cytokines and combat oxidative damage makes it one of the most effective and versatile tools for reducing chronic inflammation and promoting long-term healing.

The Role of Inflammatory Cytokines in Chronic Disease

Cytokines are small signaling proteins released by immune cells to regulate inflammation, healing, and immune responses. While some cytokines are beneficial, helping the body fight infections and repair tissue damage, others—pro-inflammatory cytokines—can become overactive, leading to excessive inflammation that harms the body instead of protecting it.

The most damaging pro-inflammatory cytokines include:

- **Tumor Necrosis Factor-alpha (TNF-α):** A major driver of chronic inflammation, TNF-α is elevated in conditions such as rheumatoid arthritis, psoriasis, Crohn's disease, and multiple sclerosis.
- **Interleukin-6 (IL-6):** High levels of IL-6 are associated with chronic pain, cardiovascular disease, and neurodegeneration.
- **Interleukin-1 beta (IL-1β):** IL-1β is a key factor in joint destruction, autoimmune flare-ups, and prolonged inflammatory responses.

When these cytokines remain active for too long, they contribute to tissue destruction, pain, and disease progression. Controlling their activity is crucial for preventing chronic illness and supporting the body's natural healing process.

How DMSO Regulates and Lowers Inflammatory Cytokines

DMSO has been scientifically shown to inhibit the overproduction of pro-inflammatory cytokines while still allowing the immune system to function properly. It does this through:

- **Blocking the release of TNF-α and IL-6:** By suppressing these key inflammatory messengers, DMSO reduces swelling, joint damage, and systemic inflammation.
- **Preventing excessive immune activation:** Many autoimmune diseases involve the immune system attacking the body's own tissues. DMSO helps balance immune responses, preventing unnecessary inflammation without completely shutting down immune function.
- **Enhancing cellular detoxification:** Chronic inflammation leads to the buildup of damaging metabolic byproducts, which further drive inflammatory processes. DMSO flushes out these toxins, reducing long-term inflammatory stress.

DMSO as a Potent Free Radical Scavenger

In addition to modulating inflammatory cytokines, DMSO is also a highly effective antioxidant, meaning it neutralizes free radicals—unstable molecules that cause oxidative damage to cells, proteins, and DNA.

Free radical damage, also known as oxidative stress, is a major contributor to aging, inflammation, and chronic disease. Some of the most harmful free radicals include:

- **Reactive Oxygen Species (ROS):** These molecules attack cell membranes, contributing to neurodegenerative diseases, cardiovascular damage, and joint degradation.
- **Nitric Oxide (NO) Overproduction:** While nitric oxide has some beneficial functions, excessive levels can lead to cellular dysfunction and inflammatory conditions.

DMSO directly scavenges and neutralizes these free radicals, preventing them from damaging cells and accelerating inflammation. Unlike synthetic antioxidants, which often have limited bioavailability, DMSO penetrates deep into tissues, reaching affected areas faster and more effectively.

By simultaneously reducing inflammatory cytokines and neutralizing oxidative stress, DMSO acts as a powerful anti-inflammatory and cellular protector, helping the body combat chronic inflammation at its core and restore optimal immune balance.

CHAPTER 8

DMSO PROTOCOLS FOR INFLAMMATORY CONDITIONS

Treating Rheumatoid Arthritis, Tendonitis, and Gout

Chronic inflammatory conditions like rheumatoid arthritis, tendonitis, and gout are often painful, debilitating, and difficult to manage with conventional treatments alone. While medications such as NSAIDs, corticosteroids, and disease-modifying anti-rheumatic drugs (DMARDs) are commonly prescribed, they often come with significant side effects and fail to address the root causes of inflammation.

DMSO stands out as a powerful natural alternative due to its anti-inflammatory, pain-relieving, and tissue-repairing properties. By penetrating deep into tissues, modulating immune responses, and improving circulation, DMSO offers relief for those struggling with persistent joint pain, stiffness, and swelling.

DMSO for Rheumatoid Arthritis: Controlling Autoimmune Inflammation

Rheumatoid arthritis (RA) is an autoimmune disorder in which the immune system mistakenly attacks the synovial lining of the joints, leading to chronic inflammation, pain, and joint deformity over time. The persistent swelling and immune activation result in cartilage erosion and reduced mobility, making RA one of the most challenging forms of arthritis to manage.

DMSO offers several key benefits for RA sufferers:

- **Regulating immune system overactivity:** Unlike corticosteroids, which suppress immune function entirely, DMSO modulates immune responses, preventing excessive inflammation without compromising overall immunity.
- **Reducing joint swelling and stiffness:** By blocking pro-inflammatory cytokines such as TNF-α and IL-6, DMSO helps prevent joint damage and pain flare-ups.
- **Improving blood circulation in affected joints:** Poor blood flow is a common issue in RA, limiting nutrient delivery and tissue repair. DMSO enhances microcirculation, ensuring that damaged cartilage and synovial tissues receive adequate oxygen and nutrients for healing.

By incorporating DMSO into a holistic RA treatment protocol, patients may experience reduced pain, improved mobility, and fewer disease flare-ups, allowing them to regain control over their daily lives.

DMSO for Tendonitis: Accelerating Recovery from Overuse Injuries

Tendonitis is a painful inflammation of the tendons, often caused by overuse, repetitive strain, or sports injuries. It commonly affects areas such as the shoulders, elbows, wrists, and Achilles tendon, leading to swelling, stiffness, and reduced range of motion.

DMSO is particularly effective for tendonitis recovery due to its ability to:

- **Reduce inflammation at the source:** Unlike oral painkillers, which take time to act, DMSO penetrates directly into the inflamed tendon, providing targeted relief.
- **Enhance tendon flexibility and strength:** Chronic inflammation weakens tendons over time, increasing the risk of ruptures and long-term damage. DMSO improves collagen production, supporting proper tendon regeneration.
- **Speed up the repair process:** By improving oxygenation and waste removal, DMSO helps tendons heal faster, allowing individuals to return to normal activities without prolonged downtime.

This makes DMSO a valuable addition to tendonitis recovery, especially for athletes, individuals with physically demanding jobs, and those prone to repetitive strain injuries.

DMSO for Gout: Reducing Uric Acid Crystals and Joint Inflammation

Gout is a metabolic inflammatory condition caused by high uric acid levels, which form sharp, needle-like crystals in the joints. These crystals trigger intense pain, swelling, and redness, primarily affecting the big toe, ankles, and knees.

DMSO can play a crucial role in managing gout attacks and preventing long-term joint damage by:

- **Reducing inflammation and pain:** DMSO blocks inflammatory pathways responsible for gout flare-ups, providing rapid relief.
- **Dissolving uric acid buildup:** Some studies suggest that DMSO improves uric acid solubility, helping the body eliminate excess deposits more efficiently.
- **Enhancing joint mobility and function:** Gout attacks often leave joints feeling stiff and weakened. DMSO improves circulation and promotes tissue hydration, restoring joint flexibility after an acute episode.

By incorporating DMSO into gout management strategies, individuals may experience fewer flare-ups, reduced joint damage, and improved long-term mobility.

DMSO's ability to penetrate tissues, control inflammation, and promote healing makes it an exceptional therapeutic option for those suffering from rheumatoid arthritis, tendonitis, and gout, offering a safe, science-backed alternative to conventional treatments.

DMSO Combinations: Using MSM, Turmeric, and Omega-3s for Maximum Effect

While DMSO is highly effective on its own, its therapeutic potential is significantly enhanced when combined with other natural anti-inflammatory compounds. Three of the most synergistic substances that work alongside DMSO are MSM (methylsulfonylmethane), turmeric, and omega-3 fatty acids. Each of these ingredients offers unique benefits, but when used together, they create a powerful, multi-layered approach to combating inflammation, reducing pain, and promoting long-term healing.

MSM and DMSO: A Sulfur-Based Synergy

MSM, a naturally occurring organosulfur compound, is often used for joint health, tissue repair, and inflammation control. It shares a similar molecular structure with DMSO and is known for its ability to enhance cellular permeability, improve collagen production, and detoxify the body.

When combined with DMSO, MSM amplifies its anti-inflammatory properties by:

- **Enhancing tissue penetration:** MSM allows DMSO to carry more nutrients and active compounds into cells, improving their bioavailability.
- **Supporting joint and cartilage health:** MSM helps rebuild damaged cartilage, reducing joint stiffness and improving flexibility.
- **Detoxifying cells:** Both DMSO and MSM aid in removing heavy metals and oxidative waste, reducing toxic burden on the body.

Many individuals struggling with arthritis, fibromyalgia, or sports injuries find that combining MSM with DMSO leads to faster pain relief and longer-lasting results, particularly for joint and connective tissue conditions.

Turmeric and DMSO: A Potent Anti-Inflammatory Duo

Turmeric, specifically its active compound curcumin, is one of the most extensively studied natural anti-inflammatory agents. It works by blocking NF-κB, a key molecular driver of chronic inflammation, and reducing levels of pro-inflammatory cytokines such as TNF-α and IL-6.

When used in combination with DMSO, turmeric becomes even more powerful due to:

- **Enhanced absorption:** Curcumin is notoriously difficult for the body to absorb. DMSO helps transport curcumin deep into tissues, ensuring greater bioavailability and effectiveness.
- **Reduction in systemic inflammation:** While DMSO is excellent for localized pain relief, turmeric provides whole-body anti-inflammatory effects, addressing conditions like autoimmune disorders and chronic inflammatory diseases.
- **Joint and muscle support:** Curcumin's ability to reduce oxidative stress and inhibit inflammatory enzymes makes it a valuable addition for those dealing with arthritis, muscle pain, and post-injury recovery.

By pairing DMSO with turmeric, individuals experience greater relief from inflammation-related pain, particularly for conditions such as rheumatoid arthritis, tendonitis, and post-surgical recovery.

Omega-3 Fatty Acids and DMSO: Reducing Inflammation at a Cellular Level

Omega-3 fatty acids, found in fish oil, flaxseed, and walnuts, are essential for reducing chronic inflammation and improving overall cellular function. These healthy fats are integral to brain health, cardiovascular function, and joint lubrication.

When combined with DMSO, omega-3s:

- **Reduce systemic inflammation:** Omega-3s lower pro-inflammatory prostaglandins, helping to relieve joint pain, stiffness, and swelling.
- **Protect against oxidative stress:** Like DMSO, omega-3s combat free radicals, reducing tissue damage and accelerating healing.
- **Improve cell membrane function:** Healthy cell membranes are essential for nutrient absorption and waste elimination. DMSO enhances cellular uptake of omega-3s, optimizing their effectiveness.

For those suffering from chronic pain conditions, cardiovascular issues, or metabolic disorders, combining DMSO with omega-3 fatty acids provides a comprehensive anti-inflammatory strategy that works from both inside and outside the body.

By combining DMSO with MSM, turmeric, and omega-3s, individuals can experience a more powerful and sustained reduction in inflammation, improving joint health, muscle recovery, and overall well-being in a way that conventional treatments often fail to achieve.

BOOK 5
DMSO FOR JOINT AND MUSCLE HEALTH

CHAPTER 9
STRENGTHENING JOINTS AND PREVENTING DEGENERATION

Rebuilding Cartilage with DMSO and Supporting Nutrients

Cartilage is the flexible, shock-absorbing tissue that cushions joints, allowing for smooth and pain-free movement. Over time, due to aging, inflammation, injury, or chronic conditions like osteoarthritis, cartilage can wear down, leading to joint stiffness, discomfort, and reduced mobility. Unlike other tissues, cartilage has a limited ability to regenerate, making joint degeneration a major cause of chronic pain and disability.

DMSO offers a powerful, science-backed approach to supporting cartilage repair. Unlike conventional treatments that only manage symptoms, DMSO penetrates deeply into tissues, reduces inflammation, enhances nutrient absorption, and stimulates cartilage regeneration. When paired with key supporting nutrients, it creates an optimal environment for joint healing, providing long-term relief from pain and stiffness.

How DMSO Supports Cartilage Regeneration

DMSO works at a cellular level, targeting the root causes of cartilage deterioration rather than simply masking pain. Its regenerative effects come from its ability to:

- **Improve chondrocyte function:** Chondrocytes are the specialized cells responsible for cartilage production and maintenance. DMSO helps these cells function more efficiently, promoting the formation of new cartilage matrix.
- **Enhance blood flow to joint tissues:** Cartilage lacks direct blood supply, making it difficult for nutrients and oxygen to reach damaged areas. DMSO improves circulation in surrounding tissues, ensuring that essential nutrients reach cartilage cells for proper regeneration.
- **Reduce oxidative stress:** Free radicals contribute to cartilage breakdown and accelerate joint degeneration. DMSO acts as a potent antioxidant, neutralizing oxidative damage and preserving joint health.
- **Modulate inflammation:** Chronic inflammation destroys cartilage over time. DMSO blocks inflammatory cytokines like TNF-α and IL-6, preventing the degradation of joint tissues.

By directly influencing cartilage repair mechanisms, DMSO provides long-term benefits for those suffering from degenerative joint conditions, helping to slow down the progression of osteoarthritis and improve joint flexibility.

Essential Nutrients for Cartilage Repair

While DMSO enhances cartilage regeneration, its effects are amplified when combined with nutrients that support joint health. These include:

- **Glucosamine and Chondroitin:** These compounds are building blocks of cartilage, essential for maintaining joint cushioning and lubrication. When absorbed efficiently, they help slow cartilage breakdown and promote repair.
- **MSM (Methylsulfonylmethane):** A natural sulfur compound that works synergistically with DMSO, MSM supports collagen production, reduces joint inflammation, and enhances flexibility.
- **Collagen Peptides:** Collagen provides the structural framework for cartilage, helping to strengthen joints and improve elasticity. DMSO enhances collagen absorption, ensuring that damaged tissues receive adequate support.
- **Hyaluronic Acid:** A key component of synovial fluid, hyaluronic acid helps keep joints lubricated, preventing friction and further cartilage erosion.
- **Vitamin C:** Essential for collagen synthesis, vitamin C plays a critical role in cartilage repair and protection from oxidative damage.

The Combined Power of DMSO and Nutrients

DMSO acts as a delivery system, carrying glucosamine, MSM, collagen, and other essential nutrients deep into joint tissues, ensuring maximum absorption and effectiveness. This unique combination allows for:

- **Faster cartilage regeneration:** Nutrients reach damaged joint structures more efficiently, supporting new tissue formation.
- **Reduced joint stiffness and improved mobility:** As cartilage regenerates, joints regain their natural flexibility and range of motion.
- **Long-term protection against degeneration:** By maintaining healthy cartilage, individuals experience less pain, greater joint stability, and long-lasting relief.

DMSO, combined with targeted nutrients, provides an effective, science-backed strategy for rebuilding cartilage, preventing further joint damage, and restoring mobility, making it an essential part of natural joint care protocols.

Long-Term Use of DMSO for Osteoarthritis Management

Osteoarthritis is a progressive degenerative joint disease that affects millions of people worldwide. Unlike acute injuries, which heal over time, osteoarthritis gradually wears down the protective cartilage in joints, leading to chronic pain, stiffness, and loss of mobility. Conventional treatments, such as NSAIDs, corticosteroids, and joint replacement surgery, offer only temporary relief or invasive solutions, failing to address the underlying degeneration of joint structures.

DMSO has emerged as a powerful, natural alternative for managing osteoarthritis in the long term.

Unlike pharmaceutical treatments that only mask pain, DMSO works at the cellular level, offering anti-inflammatory, cartilage-protective, and pain-modulating effects that support joint function and slow disease progression.

Modulating Inflammation to Prevent Joint Degradation

Chronic inflammation plays a key role in osteoarthritis progression. The breakdown of cartilage triggers an inflammatory response, leading to the release of cytokines and enzymes that further degrade joint tissues. This cycle of inflammation and destruction accelerates joint deterioration, making pain and stiffness worse over time.

DMSO effectively interrupts this process by:

- **Reducing inflammatory cytokines:** DMSO inhibits TNF-α, IL-6, and prostaglandins, which are responsible for joint inflammation and pain.
- **Suppressing oxidative stress:** Free radicals contribute to cartilage breakdown. DMSO acts as a potent antioxidant, protecting joint tissues from further degradation.
- **Preventing synovial inflammation:** The synovial membrane produces joint fluid, which keeps joints lubricated. DMSO helps maintain healthy synovial function, preventing fluid imbalance and excessive joint friction.

By controlling chronic inflammation, DMSO not only relieves pain but also slows the underlying damage responsible for osteoarthritis progression.

Protecting Cartilage and Enhancing Joint Longevity

One of the most critical aspects of long-term osteoarthritis management is protecting existing cartilage and encouraging healthy tissue regeneration. Since cartilage has limited blood supply, it heals very slowly, making preservation and repair crucial.

DMSO supports cartilage health by:

- **Enhancing chondrocyte function:** Chondrocytes are cartilage-producing cells. DMSO improves their ability to synthesize collagen and repair minor cartilage damage.
- **Delivering essential nutrients:** Many joint supplements, such as glucosamine, MSM, and hyaluronic acid, struggle with poor absorption. DMSO acts as a carrier, ensuring these nutrients reach damaged cartilage effectively.
- **Increasing hydration in joint tissues:** Cartilage relies on fluid retention for cushioning and flexibility. DMSO helps maintain proper hydration, preventing joint stiffness and fragility.

Long-Term Pain Modulation Without Dangerous Side Effects

Chronic osteoarthritis pain is often managed with painkillers, but long-term use of NSAIDs and opioids can lead to digestive issues, cardiovascular risks, and addiction. DMSO provides a safer alternative by:

- **Blocking nerve pain transmission:** DMSO interferes with pain signaling at the nerve level, providing natural analgesic effects.

- **Preventing stiffness-related discomfort:** By reducing joint swelling and improving flexibility, DMSO helps keep joints more mobile and functional over time.
- **Supporting long-term mobility:** Unlike temporary pain relief methods, regular use of DMSO helps sustain joint function, allowing individuals to remain active and independent.

Through consistent, long-term use, DMSO offers a comprehensive approach to osteoarthritis management, providing pain relief, inflammation control, and joint preservation, making it an invaluable tool for those seeking natural, effective solutions for their joint health.

CHAPTER 10
DMSO FOR MUSCLE RECOVERY AND SPORTS INJURIES

Enhancing Athletic Performance and Recovery with DMSO

Athletes constantly push their bodies to the limit, subjecting muscles, joints, and connective tissues to intense physical stress. Whether through rigorous training, competition, or repetitive movement, the demands placed on the musculoskeletal system require efficient recovery, inflammation control, and injury prevention to sustain peak performance. While traditional recovery methods, such as ice baths, massage therapy, and NSAIDs, offer some relief, they often fail to address deep tissue healing and come with limitations.

DMSO presents a unique and powerful solution for athletes looking to enhance performance, speed up muscle recovery, and reduce injury risk. By penetrating deep into tissues, reducing oxidative stress, and promoting cellular repair, DMSO offers a scientifically backed approach to maximizing athletic potential while minimizing downtime.

Reducing Exercise-Induced Inflammation for Faster Recovery

Intense physical activity leads to microtrauma in muscle fibers, which triggers inflammation and soreness as the body initiates the repair process. While inflammation is a necessary part of muscle adaptation, excessive or prolonged inflammation delays recovery, increases stiffness, and raises the risk of overuse injuries.

DMSO helps regulate this inflammatory response by:

- **Inhibiting pro-inflammatory cytokines:** Excessive production of TNF-α, IL-6, and prostaglandins leads to prolonged muscle soreness and joint stiffness. DMSO modulates these inflammatory signals, reducing post-exercise discomfort.
- **Enhancing blood circulation and nutrient delivery:** Efficient blood flow is crucial for removing metabolic waste (lactic acid) and delivering oxygen to fatigued muscles. DMSO improves microvascular circulation, expediting the body's natural recovery process.
- **Reducing swelling in overworked muscles:** By preventing excessive fluid accumulation, DMSO helps muscles recover faster and with less discomfort, allowing athletes to return to training sooner.

Unlike NSAIDs, which merely suppress pain and inflammation, DMSO actively supports healing, making it a safer, long-term solution for managing post-exercise recovery.

Preventing Muscle Fatigue and Enhancing Endurance

Muscle fatigue occurs when cells struggle to produce enough energy to sustain prolonged activity. The buildup of oxidative stress, lactic acid, and inflammatory byproducts further impairs muscle function, reducing strength, endurance, and overall performance.

DMSO combats muscle fatigue by:

- **Neutralizing free radicals:** Intense exercise generates reactive oxygen species (ROS), which accelerate muscle breakdown and slow recovery. DMSO scavenges free radicals, protecting muscle cells from oxidative damage.
- **Improving mitochondrial function:** Mitochondria are the energy-producing structures in cells. DMSO enhances oxygen utilization and ATP production, allowing muscles to sustain higher levels of performance for longer durations.
- **Supporting electrolyte balance:** Muscle cramps and spasms are often caused by electrolyte imbalances. DMSO facilitates cellular hydration, reducing the likelihood of fatigue-related muscle contractions.

By protecting muscles from oxidative damage and improving energy efficiency, DMSO enhances endurance, allowing athletes to train harder, longer, and more effectively.

Minimizing Injury Risk and Supporting Tissue Regeneration

Athletes are at high risk for muscle strains, ligament sprains, and joint injuries, which can sideline them for weeks or even months. A critical part of any athletic program is not just recovery but also injury prevention. DMSO helps maintain muscle, tendon, and joint integrity, reducing the risk of long-term damage.

DMSO plays a crucial role in injury prevention and tissue repair by:

- **Strengthening connective tissues:** DMSO enhances collagen production, improving the elasticity and resilience of tendons and ligaments.
- **Preventing scar tissue formation:** After injuries, excessive scar tissue reduces flexibility and increases re-injury risk. DMSO helps break down fibrotic adhesions, ensuring proper healing with minimal stiffness.
- **Supporting joint lubrication:** Healthy cartilage and synovial fluid are essential for smooth, pain-free movement. DMSO improves joint hydration and reduces friction, preserving long-term joint function.

For athletes looking to optimize performance, accelerate recovery, and prevent injuries, DMSO provides a natural, science-backed advantage, ensuring stronger, healthier muscles and joints over time.

Treating Ligament and Tendon Damage for Faster Healing

Ligaments and tendons are critical connective tissues that provide stability and movement to joints and muscles. However, due to overuse, high-impact activities, or sudden injuries, these structures are prone to tears, strains, and inflammation. Unlike muscles, which have a rich blood supply and heal relatively quickly, ligaments and tendons have limited circulation, making their recovery slow and challenging.

DMSO has gained attention as a highly effective natural therapy for accelerating ligament and tendon repair. With its deep tissue penetration, anti-inflammatory properties, and ability to enhance cellular regeneration, DMSO offers a powerful alternative to conventional treatments that often involve painkillers, corticosteroids, or prolonged physical therapy.

How Ligament and Tendon Injuries Occur

Ligaments connect bone to bone, providing joint stability, while tendons connect muscles to bones, allowing for movement and force transmission. When exposed to excessive strain, repetitive motion, or sudden impact, these connective tissues can become inflamed, overstretched, or torn, leading to pain, swelling, and limited mobility.

Common ligament and tendon injuries include:

- **Sprains:** Overstretching or tearing of a ligament, commonly affecting the ankle, knee, or wrist.
- **Tendonitis:** Inflammation of a tendon due to repetitive motion, seen frequently in the shoulder (rotator cuff), elbow (tennis elbow), and Achilles tendon.
- **Tendon tears:** Partial or complete rupture of a tendon, often occurring in the Achilles tendon, patellar tendon, or biceps tendon.

Because these tissues are slow to regenerate, injuries often require extended recovery periods, leaving individuals unable to train, work, or engage in physical activities.

How DMSO Enhances Ligament and Tendon Healing

DMSO accelerates the repair process for ligament and tendon injuries by targeting inflammation, enhancing collagen production, and improving nutrient delivery to damaged tissues.

- **Reduces Inflammatory Damage:** Inflammation in ligaments and tendons often leads to stiffness, swelling, and prolonged recovery time. DMSO inhibits pro-inflammatory cytokines such as TNF-α and IL-6, reducing pain and tissue breakdown.
- **Improves Collagen Synthesis:** Collagen is the structural protein responsible for tendon and ligament strength. DMSO stimulates fibroblast activity, encouraging the production of new collagen fibers to repair damaged connective tissue.
- **Prevents Scar Tissue Formation:** When ligaments or tendons heal improperly, excessive scar tissue can form, leading to restricted mobility and increased re-injury risk. DMSO prevents fibrotic buildup, ensuring strong, flexible tissue repair.
- **Enhances Blood Flow and Nutrient Absorption:** The limited circulation in ligaments and tendons slows down healing, but DMSO improves microvascular circulation, ensuring oxygen and essential nutrients reach damaged areas for faster recovery.

Preventing Re-Injury and Strengthening Connective Tissues

One of the biggest challenges after a ligament or tendon injury is preventing recurrence. Weak or improperly healed connective tissues are more prone to re-injury, which can lead to chronic instability and long-term functional issues.

DMSO plays a key role in preventing future injuries by:

- **Restoring tissue elasticity:** Unlike some treatments that focus only on pain relief, DMSO helps ligaments and tendons regain flexibility and tensile strength.
- **Enhancing cellular hydration:** Proper hydration is essential for keeping connective tissues pliable and resistant to tearing.
- **Reducing oxidative stress:** Repeated injuries create oxidative damage, weakening connective structures. DMSO neutralizes free radicals, protecting tendons and ligaments from degeneration.

By incorporating DMSO into ligament and tendon recovery protocols, individuals can heal faster, strengthen their connective tissues, and return to physical activity with reduced risk of long-term complications.

BOOK 6
DMSO FOR SKIN CONDITIONS AND WOUND HEALING

CHAPTER 11
THE SKIN-REJUVENATING POWER OF DMSO

Treating Burns, Cuts, and Ulcers with DMSO Applications

The skin is the body's first line of defense, protecting against infections, environmental toxins, and physical injuries. However, burns, cuts, and ulcers can compromise this barrier, leading to pain, inflammation, and an increased risk of infection. Proper wound care is essential to prevent complications and accelerate healing, but conventional treatments often focus solely on symptom management, rather than enhancing tissue repair at a cellular level.

DMSO is an exceptionally powerful natural agent for treating skin injuries, offering anti-inflammatory, antimicrobial, and regenerative properties. Unlike traditional topical treatments that act only on the surface, DMSO penetrates deep into tissues, promoting faster wound healing, reducing scarring, and preventing infection.

Accelerating Burn Recovery and Reducing Pain

Burns, whether caused by heat, chemicals, or friction, lead to cellular damage, fluid loss, and inflammation. Severe burns can result in long-term scarring and impaired skin function, making rapid tissue regeneration crucial for recovery.

DMSO's effectiveness in burn treatment comes from its ability to:

- **Reduce pain and inflammation:** Burns trigger intense inflammatory responses, leading to swelling and nerve sensitivity. DMSO blocks pro-inflammatory cytokines, alleviating pain and discomfort within minutes.
- **Prevent blister formation:** The fluid buildup that leads to blisters can prolong healing and increase infection risks. DMSO improves microcirculation, reducing fluid retention and promoting faster skin regeneration.
- **Protect against oxidative damage:** Burns generate free radicals, which accelerate tissue destruction. DMSO acts as a powerful antioxidant, neutralizing these harmful molecules and preserving healthy skin cells.

By modulating the inflammatory response and promoting rapid cell regeneration, DMSO enhances skin recovery, minimizing long-term damage and scarring.

Wound Healing: Faster Tissue Repair for Cuts and Lacerations

Cuts and lacerations expose the underlying tissues to bacteria and environmental contaminants, increasing the risk of infection and prolonged healing. The natural clotting and scab formation process is crucial, but inefficient healing can lead to excessive scarring or slow tissue regeneration.

DMSO accelerates wound healing by:

- **Stimulating fibroblast activity:** Fibroblasts are the key cells responsible for tissue repair and collagen synthesis. DMSO enhances their function, ensuring stronger, healthier skin regeneration.
- **Enhancing blood flow to the wound site:** Efficient circulation is essential for delivering oxygen and nutrients necessary for new skin formation. DMSO improves vascular function, promoting faster healing and reduced scarring.
- **Preventing bacterial infections:** Unlike conventional antiseptics, which only work at the surface, DMSO penetrates deep into tissues, carrying antimicrobial agents into the wound to prevent bacterial growth and sepsis.

These properties make DMSO an essential tool for treating cuts and open wounds, ensuring cleaner, faster healing while minimizing the risk of scarring and infection.

Ulcer Treatment: Breaking the Cycle of Chronic Wound Formation

Chronic ulcers—such as pressure sores, diabetic ulcers, and venous ulcers—develop when skin and tissue break down due to poor circulation, prolonged inflammation, or infection. Unlike minor wounds, ulcers struggle to heal naturally, making effective intervention crucial.

DMSO supports ulcer recovery by:

- **Reducing chronic inflammation:** Persistent inflammation prevents proper tissue repair. DMSO blocks inflammatory enzymes, allowing ulcers to transition from an inflamed state to an active healing phase.
- **Improving tissue oxygenation:** Oxygen delivery is essential for new skin cell growth, but many ulcer patients suffer from poor circulation. DMSO enhances capillary function, ensuring sufficient oxygen supply to damaged tissues.
- **Breaking down biofilms:** Chronic ulcers often develop bacterial biofilms, which make them resistant to traditional treatments. DMSO disrupts bacterial colonies, promoting faster healing and infection control.

By targeting the root causes of ulcer formation—poor circulation, inflammation, and infection—DMSO helps break the cycle of chronic wounds, promoting effective skin regeneration where other treatments fail.

Using DMSO for Chronic Skin Conditions: Eczema, Psoriasis, and Dermatitis

Chronic skin conditions such as eczema, psoriasis, and dermatitis affect millions of people, causing persistent itching, redness, inflammation, and discomfort. While conventional treatments—such as steroid creams, antihistamines, and immunosuppressants—can provide temporary relief, they often fail to address the underlying causes of skin inflammation and may lead to long-term side effects.

DMSO presents a powerful natural alternative for individuals seeking effective, science-backed solutions for chronic skin conditions. With its deep tissue penetration, anti-inflammatory properties, and ability to modulate immune responses, DMSO offers relief from symptoms while actively repairing damaged skin and restoring balance to the body's inflammatory pathways.

Eczema: Restoring the Skin Barrier and Reducing Flare-Ups

Eczema, also known as atopic dermatitis, is characterized by dry, inflamed, and itchy skin that often worsens due to triggers such as allergens, stress, and climate changes. One of the primary causes of eczema is a compromised skin barrier, which allows irritants and pathogens to penetrate, leading to chronic inflammation and itching cycles.

DMSO helps individuals with eczema by:

- **Reducing skin inflammation:** By blocking inflammatory cytokines like IL-6 and TNF-α, DMSO helps soothe red, swollen, and irritated skin.
- **Restoring the skin's protective barrier:** Unlike conventional creams that sit on the surface, DMSO penetrates deep into the skin, helping retain moisture and repair the epidermis.
- **Providing anti-itch relief:** Many eczema sufferers struggle with persistent itchiness, which leads to scratching, wounds, and infections. DMSO helps calm overactive nerve endings, reducing the urge to scratch.

By addressing both inflammation and skin barrier dysfunction, DMSO can help reduce eczema flare-ups and promote long-term skin resilience.

Psoriasis: Modulating the Immune Response to Prevent Scaling and Inflammation

Psoriasis is an autoimmune-driven skin disorder in which the immune system mistakenly accelerates skin cell production, leading to thick, scaly patches, inflammation, and discomfort. Traditional psoriasis treatments focus on immune suppression, but this approach often comes with significant side effects and limited long-term success.

DMSO is particularly effective for psoriasis because it:

- **Modulates the immune system:** Instead of suppressing immune function completely, DMSO helps balance hyperactive immune responses, reducing skin cell overproduction and inflammatory flare-ups.
- **Softens and removes plaques:** Psoriasis plaques consist of thickened, hardened skin cells that cause discomfort and flaking. DMSO penetrates plaques, loosening dead skin layers, and allowing for gentler exfoliation.
- **Reduces oxidative stress:** Free radicals contribute to psoriasis flare-ups and skin damage. DMSO acts as a powerful antioxidant, preventing further skin deterioration and supporting cellular regeneration.

With regular use, DMSO can help individuals with psoriasis manage symptoms more effectively, reduce plaque formation, and restore skin smoothness.

Dermatitis: Calming Irritated and Hypersensitive Skin

Dermatitis is an umbrella term for various forms of skin irritation, including contact dermatitis, seborrheic dermatitis, and allergic reactions. Many cases of dermatitis are triggered by external irritants, environmental toxins, or overactive immune responses, leading to red, inflamed, and peeling skin.

DMSO provides relief for dermatitis by:

- **Neutralizing allergens and irritants:** DMSO binds to and flushes out chemical irritants, preventing prolonged skin inflammation.
- **Improving circulation to damaged skin:** Enhanced blood flow ensures faster delivery of nutrients and oxygen, helping the skin heal more efficiently.
- **Reducing skin hypersensitivity:** Many dermatitis sufferers experience skin reactivity to soaps, fragrances, and fabrics. DMSO strengthens the skin's resilience, making it less prone to future irritation.

By addressing both the root causes and symptoms of chronic skin conditions, DMSO offers a safe, natural, and highly effective approach to managing eczema, psoriasis, and dermatitis, helping individuals achieve clearer, healthier skin without dependency on pharmaceutical treatments.

CHAPTER 12
ANTI-AGING AND COSMETIC BENEFITS OF DMSO

DIY DMSO-Based Skin Serums for a Youthful Glow

A radiant, youthful complexion is the ultimate goal for those seeking natural skincare solutions. While many commercial anti-aging products promise miraculous results, they often contain harsh chemicals, artificial preservatives, and synthetic fillers that provide only temporary effects. DMSO, on the other hand, is a science-backed, deeply penetrating compound that enhances skin health at a cellular level, promoting hydration, elasticity, and collagen regeneration.

By incorporating DMSO-based skin serums into a regular skincare routine, individuals can maximize the benefits of natural anti-aging ingredients, ensuring that nutrients penetrate deeper into the skin for visible, long-lasting results.

Why DMSO is the Perfect Base for Skin Serums

Unlike traditional serums that only work at the surface, DMSO acts as a delivery system, carrying active ingredients deep into the skin layers where they can exert maximum rejuvenating effects. This makes DMSO a unique and powerful addition to any anti-aging skincare formula.

The key reasons why DMSO is an ideal base for DIY skin serums include:

- **Deep tissue penetration:** DMSO transports collagen-boosting and hydrating ingredients beyond the outer epidermis, ensuring faster and more effective skin renewal.
- **Anti-inflammatory properties:** Many skin concerns, including redness, irritation, and premature aging, stem from chronic inflammation. DMSO calms overactive inflammatory responses, leading to a clearer, healthier complexion.
- **Antioxidant activity:** Free radicals contribute to wrinkles, sagging, and dull skin tone. DMSO neutralizes oxidative stress, protecting skin from pollution, UV exposure, and environmental toxins.
- **Increased hydration retention:** By strengthening the skin's moisture barrier, DMSO prevents water loss, ensuring that skin stays plump, firm, and youthful.

Key Ingredients to Pair with DMSO for Maximum Benefits

While DMSO works exceptionally well on its own, combining it with potent natural ingredients enhances its rejuvenating and hydrating effects.

- **Hyaluronic Acid:** One of the most powerful humectants, hyaluronic acid locks in moisture, giving skin a dewy, plump appearance.
- **Vitamin C (Ascorbic Acid):** A potent antioxidant that brightens skin, fades dark spots, and boosts collagen production.
- **Collagen Peptides:** Supports skin elasticity and structure, reducing the appearance of fine lines and wrinkles.
- **Rosehip Oil:** Rich in essential fatty acids and vitamin A, rosehip oil helps to heal damaged skin, even out tone, and promote elasticity.
- **Aloe Vera:** Soothes and hydrates sensitive or inflamed skin, making it perfect for balancing DMSO's potency.

By combining DMSO with these targeted ingredients, DIY serums penetrate deeper, nourish more effectively, and deliver dramatic skin-enhancing results.

Enhancing Skin Health Naturally

The beauty of DMSO-based serums lies in their ability to work with the skin's natural regenerative processes. Unlike store-bought anti-aging treatments that rely on synthetic preservatives and temporary plumping agents, DMSO optimizes skin function at a cellular level, helping to:

- Reduce fine lines and wrinkles without artificial fillers.
- Improve elasticity and firmness by promoting collagen synthesis.
- Even out skin tone and reduce the appearance of sun damage.
- Restore hydration and give the skin a radiant, youthful glow.

Incorporating DMSO into a DIY skincare regimen allows individuals to experience real, long-lasting results using pure, skin-loving ingredients, free from toxic additives or unnecessary chemicals.

DIY DMSO-Based Skin Serums for a Youthful Glow

Achieving radiant, youthful skin is often seen as a complex and expensive process, filled with high-end creams, serums, and cosmetic treatments. However, many of these products contain harsh chemicals, preservatives, and synthetic fillers that offer temporary results without truly nourishing the skin. For those seeking a natural and science-backed solution, DIY DMSO-based skin serums provide an effective alternative, offering deep hydration, wrinkle reduction, and long-term skin health benefits.

Unlike traditional skincare products, DMSO penetrates the skin barrier, delivering nutrients and antioxidants directly to the deeper layers of the skin, where they can stimulate repair and rejuvenation.

When carefully formulated with complementary ingredients, DMSO-based serums nourish the skin at a cellular level, enhancing its elasticity, hydration, and overall radiance.

Why DMSO is a Game-Changer for Skin Care

DMSO is a unique compound with multiple properties that make it an ideal base for a high-performance anti-aging serum:

- **Deep tissue penetration:** Unlike conventional creams that sit on the surface, DMSO transports active ingredients deep into the dermis, where collagen production and skin regeneration take place.
- **Powerful antioxidant action:** Free radicals are a leading cause of premature aging. DMSO helps neutralize oxidative stress, protecting the skin from environmental damage and UV-related aging.
- **Anti-inflammatory properties:** Chronic inflammation contributes to skin redness, irritation, and accelerated aging. DMSO calms inflammatory responses, reducing puffiness and restoring a balanced skin tone.
- **Hydration and moisture retention:** Aging skin often loses its ability to retain moisture, leading to dullness and fine lines. DMSO helps lock in hydration, giving skin a plump, supple appearance.

Best Ingredients to Pair with DMSO for Maximum Skin Benefits

When combined with targeted natural ingredients, DMSO-based serums enhance skin renewal, reduce fine lines, and restore elasticity. Some of the most effective ingredients to include are:

- **Hyaluronic Acid:** A deeply hydrating molecule that binds moisture to the skin, keeping it firm, smooth, and plump.
- **Vitamin C (Ascorbic Acid):** A powerful antioxidant that brightens the complexion, fades dark spots, and stimulates collagen synthesis.
- **Collagen Peptides:** Boosts skin structure and firmness, reducing the appearance of sagging and wrinkles.
- **Aloe Vera Gel:** Soothes and hydrates sensitive skin, reducing redness and irritation while promoting cellular regeneration.
- **Rosehip Oil:** Rich in essential fatty acids and retinoids, it supports skin elasticity, improves tone, and reduces the visibility of scars and fine lines.

How DMSO-Based Serums Improve Skin Health Over Time

While many skincare products offer instant, superficial effects, DMSO-based serums work from within, addressing deep-rooted skin concerns at a cellular level. Over time, consistent use leads to:

- Visible reduction in wrinkles and fine lines, as skin firms and plumps naturally.
- Improved skin tone and elasticity, restoring a youthful, lifted appearance.
- Balanced hydration and reduced dryness, preventing flakiness and dullness.
- Smoother skin texture, as dead skin cells are removed faster, promoting natural renewal.

By combining DMSO with carefully selected nutrients, individuals can experience long-term skin rejuvenation, ensuring a healthy, youthful glow without the need for harsh chemicals or expensive treatments.

BOOK 7
DMSO FOR IMMUNE SUPPORT AND INFECTIONS

CHAPTER 13
FIGHTING BACTERIAL INFECTIONS WITH DMSO

Treating Staph, Cellulitis, and UTIs Naturally

Bacterial infections such as staph (Staphylococcus infections), cellulitis, and urinary tract infections (UTIs) can be painful, persistent, and in some cases, difficult to treat with conventional antibiotics alone. While modern medicine relies heavily on antibiotic therapy, the rise of antibiotic resistance has made it essential to explore alternative and complementary solutions for treating bacterial infections.

DMSO has emerged as a highly effective natural antimicrobial agent, with the ability to penetrate deeply into tissues, reduce inflammation, and enhance the body's immune response against bacterial infections. Its unique properties make it a powerful ally in fighting these conditions while reducing dependency on pharmaceutical antibiotics.

Fighting Staph Infections with DMSO

Staph infections, caused by Staphylococcus bacteria, range from mild skin infections to serious, potentially life-threatening conditions such as MRSA (methicillin-resistant Staphylococcus aureus). These infections often develop in cuts, wounds, and surgical sites, leading to swelling, redness, and pus formation. In severe cases, staph bacteria can enter the bloodstream, causing systemic infections that require immediate intervention.

DMSO offers a multi-faceted approach to treating staph infections by:

- **Directly inhibiting bacterial growth:** DMSO has natural antibacterial properties that help suppress staph colonization in infected tissues.
- **Enhancing immune cell activity:** By improving white blood cell function, DMSO helps the body naturally eliminate bacterial invaders more efficiently.
- **Reducing tissue inflammation:** Infected wounds often swell due to excessive immune responses. DMSO helps calm inflammatory reactions, promoting faster healing.
- **Increasing penetration of natural antimicrobials:** When combined with natural or pharmaceutical treatments, DMSO delivers active compounds deep into infected tissues, ensuring maximum efficacy.

For skin-based staph infections, rapid intervention is critical to prevent deeper tissue damage or the spread of infection into the bloodstream. By targeting both bacterial overgrowth and inflammatory responses, DMSO plays a vital role in natural staph infection management.

Cellulitis: Stopping the Spread of Deep Skin Infections

Cellulitis is a serious bacterial skin infection that spreads through the deep layers of the skin and soft tissues, often caused by Staphylococcus or Streptococcus bacteria. Symptoms include redness, swelling, warmth, and tenderness, with the potential for fever and systemic complications if untreated.

DMSO is particularly effective in managing cellulitis due to its ability to:

- Penetrate deep into infected tissues, targeting bacterial colonies at their source.
- Reduce pain and swelling, preventing the infection from worsening or spreading.
- Support lymphatic drainage, allowing the body to eliminate bacterial waste and toxins more effectively.
- Boost skin regeneration, helping damaged tissues recover without excessive scarring.

For those prone to recurring cellulitis or slow-healing skin infections, DMSO's anti-inflammatory and antimicrobial properties provide a natural method of controlling infection and restoring healthy skin function.

Urinary Tract Infections: A Natural Approach to Bacterial Overgrowth

Urinary tract infections (UTIs) are among the most common bacterial infections, often caused by Escherichia coli (E. coli) bacteria migrating from the digestive system to the bladder, urethra, or kidneys. Symptoms include painful urination, urgency, lower abdominal discomfort, and in severe cases, fever and kidney involvement.

DMSO plays a valuable role in UTI management by:

- Acting as a direct antimicrobial agent, helping to reduce bacterial loads in the urinary tract.
- Reducing bladder inflammation, easing pain and discomfort associated with UTIs.
- Improving circulation in urinary tissues, which accelerates healing and prevents bacterial adhesion to the bladder lining.
- Supporting immune system response, allowing the body to fight off recurring infections naturally.

Chronic or antibiotic-resistant UTIs can be incredibly frustrating and difficult to manage. By addressing both bacterial overgrowth and inflammation, DMSO provides an alternative, natural approach to restoring urinary tract health while reducing reliance on antibiotics.

Enhancing Antibiotic Efficacy with DMSO

The rise of antibiotic resistance has become a serious global health concern, making it increasingly difficult to treat bacterial infections effectively. Many antibiotics fail due to poor tissue penetration, bacterial resistance mechanisms, or an inability to eliminate biofilms—protective layers that bacteria form to shield themselves from drugs.

DMSO presents a unique and powerful solution to this problem. By acting as a penetration enhancer, anti-inflammatory agent, and bacterial disruptor, DMSO improves the effectiveness of antibiotics, ensuring that they reach infected tissues more efficiently while also reducing bacterial defenses. This makes DMSO a valuable adjunct therapy in combating infections that are otherwise difficult to treat with conventional antibiotics alone.

DMSO as a Carrier: Delivering Antibiotics Deep into Infected Tissues

One of the most significant limitations of antibiotics is their inability to reach deeply embedded infections. Many bacterial infections occur in poorly vascularized tissues, such as cartilage, joints, or abscesses, where blood circulation is limited. As a powerful solvent, DMSO carries antibiotic compounds through cell membranes, allowing them to penetrate deeper and reach infections that would otherwise remain untreated.

- **Improves drug absorption:** DMSO increases the bioavailability of antibiotics, ensuring that a higher concentration reaches the site of infection.
- **Bypasses drug resistance barriers:** Many bacteria develop resistance by pumping antibiotics out of their cells before they can take effect. DMSO helps deliver antibiotics past these bacterial defenses, improving their ability to eliminate infections.
- **Accelerates treatment time:** Because DMSO enhances drug penetration, antibiotics may work faster and more effectively, shortening the duration of infection.

This deep penetration effect is particularly beneficial for infections in bones (osteomyelitis), joints, and chronic wound infections, where standard antibiotic therapies often fail to reach therapeutic concentrations.

Disrupting Bacterial Biofilms for More Effective Treatment

Many chronic bacterial infections, including urinary tract infections, sinus infections, and skin abscesses, persist because bacteria form biofilms—slimy, protective layers that make them highly resistant to antibiotics.

DMSO is uniquely effective in breaking down bacterial biofilms, making bacteria more vulnerable to antibiotic treatment. It achieves this by:

- Dissolving biofilm structures, exposing bacteria to higher concentrations of antibiotics.
- Weakening bacterial defenses, allowing antibiotics to penetrate bacterial colonies more effectively.
- Preventing biofilm regrowth, reducing the risk of chronic and recurring infections.

By combining DMSO with antibiotic therapy, patients suffering from chronic infections may experience faster, more complete recovery, even in cases where traditional antibiotics alone have failed to produce results.

Reducing Inflammation and Tissue Damage During Treatment

Bacterial infections trigger intense inflammatory responses, leading to pain, swelling, and tissue destruction. In some cases, the inflammation caused by the immune system's attack on bacteria can be as damaging as the infection itself.

DMSO helps control excessive inflammation, allowing antibiotics to work more effectively without causing additional tissue damage. It does this by:

- Reducing inflammatory cytokines (TNF-α, IL-6, IL-1β), which contribute to swelling and pain.
- Minimizing oxidative stress, preventing tissue damage from free radicals released during infection.
- Enhancing circulation, ensuring that infected tissues receive more oxygen and nutrients to support healing.

This anti-inflammatory effect not only aids in recovery but also helps prevent complications such as scar tissue formation and chronic pain after infections resolve.

A Natural Solution for Overcoming Antibiotic Resistance

With antibiotic resistance becoming a growing threat, integrating DMSO into treatment protocols offers a natural, non-toxic approach to restoring antibiotic effectiveness. By improving drug penetration, disrupting bacterial biofilms, and controlling inflammation, DMSO provides a powerful tool for managing even the most persistent infections, ensuring that antibiotics work at their full potential.

CHAPTER 14
DMSO'S ROLE IN VIRAL AND FUNGAL INFECTIONS

Using DMSO for Herpes, Shingles, and Respiratory Viruses

Viral infections can be some of the most difficult conditions to manage, as viruses are notoriously resilient and capable of lying dormant in the body for years. Conditions such as herpes simplex (HSV-1 and HSV-2), shingles (herpes zoster), and respiratory viruses pose unique challenges, often resulting in painful outbreaks, chronic inflammation, and prolonged recovery periods. Conventional antiviral medications can suppress symptoms, but they often fail to eliminate the virus or prevent recurrent flare-ups.

DMSO offers a unique and promising alternative for managing viral infections, thanks to its deep tissue penetration, anti-inflammatory properties, and immune-modulating effects. It is particularly effective in reducing viral activity, soothing inflammation, and promoting faster healing of affected tissues.

Herpes Simplex: Reducing Outbreaks and Pain

Herpes simplex virus (HSV) is a lifelong viral infection that causes painful blisters on the mouth (HSV-1) or genitals (HSV-2). Once contracted, the virus remains in the nervous system, where it can reactivate due to stress, weakened immunity, or hormonal fluctuations. Traditional treatments, such as antiviral medications (acyclovir, valacyclovir), can help manage symptoms but do not eliminate the virus entirely.

DMSO provides several advantages for managing herpes outbreaks:

- **Inhibiting viral replication:** Research suggests that DMSO interferes with the ability of viruses to replicate, reducing the severity and frequency of outbreaks.
- **Penetrating nerve tissue:** Since herpes resides in nerve cells, DMSO's deep tissue penetration allows it to reach affected areas more effectively than conventional creams or oral medications.
- **Reducing inflammation and nerve pain:** Herpes outbreaks are often painful and irritating, but DMSO calms nerve inflammation, helping to reduce burning sensations and speed up healing.
- **Preventing scarring:** By enhancing skin regeneration, DMSO minimizes the risk of scarring from herpes lesions, leaving smoother, healthier skin after an outbreak subsides.

Many individuals dealing with recurrent herpes flare-ups find that DMSO not only shortens the duration of outbreaks but also helps prevent new episodes by supporting a balanced immune response.

Shingles: Managing Pain and Accelerating Recovery

Shingles (herpes zoster) is a reactivation of the varicella-zoster virus, the same virus responsible for chickenpox. It causes painful, blistering rashes along nerve pathways, often accompanied by severe nerve pain (postherpetic neuralgia) that can persist long after the rash has healed.

DMSO is particularly effective in the treatment of shingles due to its nerve-soothing and anti-inflammatory properties. It helps by:

- **Reducing acute nerve pain:** Shingles pain can be excruciating, but DMSO helps block pain signal transmission, providing rapid relief.
- **Preventing long-term nerve damage:** Many individuals suffer from postherpetic neuralgia, where nerve pain lingers for months or even years. DMSO helps protect nerve cells from long-term inflammation and scarring.
- **Speeding up rash healing:** The blisters associated with shingles can take weeks to heal, often leaving discoloration or scarring. DMSO promotes faster tissue regeneration, restoring skin health more quickly.
- **Boosting immune response:** Since shingles occurs when immune defenses weaken, DMSO enhances immune system function, making the body more resistant to further viral reactivation.

For individuals struggling with prolonged shingles pain or recurrent outbreaks, DMSO provides a natural, effective alternative to painkillers and conventional antiviral drugs.

Respiratory Viruses: Supporting Lung and Immune Health

Respiratory viruses, including influenza, common colds, and coronaviruses, primarily affect the lungs, airways, and immune system, leading to inflammation, mucus buildup, and prolonged fatigue. Conventional treatments often focus on symptom relief, but they do not always address underlying immune function or inflammation.

DMSO is highly beneficial for respiratory viral infections due to its:

- **Anti-inflammatory properties:** Many respiratory viruses cause lung and airway inflammation, leading to breathing difficulties and persistent coughing. DMSO helps reduce this inflammation, easing symptoms.
- **Improved oxygen transport:** Since severe viral infections can reduce oxygenation, DMSO enhances cellular oxygen delivery, supporting lung function and overall recovery.
- **Mucus-thinning effects:** Excess mucus buildup can block airways and worsen congestion. DMSO helps break down thick mucus, allowing for easier breathing and faster lung recovery.
- **Immune-modulating capabilities:** A balanced immune response is key to fighting respiratory infections without excessive inflammation. DMSO helps strengthen immunity while preventing overactive inflammatory responses.

For individuals prone to chronic respiratory infections, incorporating DMSO into immune-support protocols may help reduce symptom severity, improve lung function, and speed up overall recovery.

Treating Candida and Other Fungal Overgrowths

Fungal infections are persistent, difficult to eliminate, and often misdiagnosed, making them one of the most frustrating conditions to treat. Candida overgrowth, athlete's foot, nail fungus, and systemic fungal infections can cause chronic discomfort, immune dysfunction, and long-term health complications if left unaddressed. Traditional antifungal medications are frequently prescribed, but many strains of fungi have developed resistance to pharmaceutical treatments, leading to recurring infections and incomplete healing.

DMSO provides a powerful and natural approach to tackling fungal overgrowth by penetrating deep into tissues, disrupting fungal colonies, and supporting immune function. Its ability to act as a carrier for antifungal agents makes it particularly useful in breaking down biofilms and eliminating infections at the source.

Understanding Candida Overgrowth and Its Impact on the Body

Candida is a type of yeast that naturally exists in the body, particularly in the digestive tract, mouth, and vaginal flora. In a healthy individual, Candida levels remain balanced, thanks to probiotic bacteria and a strong immune system. However, factors such as high sugar diets, antibiotic overuse, chronic stress, and weakened immunity can cause Candida to overgrow, leading to digestive issues, brain fog, fatigue, and skin conditions.

Symptoms of Candida overgrowth include:

- Persistent bloating, gas, and digestive discomfort
- Unexplained fatigue and brain fog
- Recurring yeast infections or oral thrush
- Skin rashes, eczema, or fungal nail infections
- Sugar cravings and difficulty digesting carbohydrates

How DMSO Combats Candida and Other Fungal Infections

DMSO offers a multi-faceted approach to treating Candida overgrowth and fungal infections by:

- **Penetrating fungal biofilms:** Many fungal species, including Candida, form protective biofilms that shield them from antifungal treatments. DMSO disrupts these biofilms, allowing antifungal agents to reach and destroy fungal colonies.
- **Transporting antifungal compounds deeper into tissues:** Unlike many topical or oral antifungals that struggle to reach fungal infections embedded in tissues, DMSO enhances absorption and delivers antifungal agents directly to the infection site.

- **Neutralizing mycotoxins:** Fungal infections release toxins that cause inflammation, brain fog, and immune suppression. DMSO helps neutralize mycotoxins, reducing systemic symptoms.
- **Reducing inflammation and irritation:** Fungal overgrowth often leads to redness, swelling, and itching. DMSO's natural anti-inflammatory properties help soothe discomfort while allowing the body to heal.

Addressing Systemic and Surface Fungal Infections

While Candida often presents as a gut-related imbalance, fungal infections can also affect the skin, nails, and respiratory system. DMSO effectively supports the treatment of:

- **Athlete's foot and fungal skin infections:** DMSO penetrates deep into the skin layers, targeting the root cause of fungal infections, rather than just the surface symptoms.
- **Nail fungus:** Many antifungal treatments struggle to reach the nail bed, but DMSO enhances absorption, helping to eliminate fungal colonies from within.
- **Sinus and respiratory fungal infections:** Some individuals suffer from chronic sinus congestion and lung issues caused by fungal spores. DMSO assists in breaking down fungal mucus buildup and improving respiratory function.

By addressing both the symptoms and root causes of fungal infections, DMSO provides a comprehensive, natural alternative to conventional antifungal treatments, making it an effective solution for individuals dealing with persistent or resistant fungal overgrowth.

BOOK 8
DMSO FOR AUTOIMMUNE DISORDERS

CHAPTER 15
BALANCING THE IMMUNE SYSTEM WITH DMSO

How DMSO Regulates Overactive Immune Responses

The immune system is designed to protect the body from infections, toxins, and cellular abnormalities, but when it becomes overactive or dysregulated, it can lead to chronic inflammation, allergic reactions, and autoimmune diseases. Many conditions, such as rheumatoid arthritis, lupus, multiple sclerosis, and inflammatory bowel disease, stem from an immune system that mistakenly attacks healthy tissues. Conventional treatments often rely on immunosuppressant drugs, which can weaken the body's ability to fight infections and come with serious long-term side effects.

DMSO offers a unique alternative by helping to balance immune function rather than simply suppressing it. With its anti-inflammatory, antioxidant, and immune-modulating properties, DMSO can help individuals regulate immune overactivity, providing relief from chronic inflammation and immune dysfunction without compromising overall immune defense.

Modulating Inflammatory Cytokines to Prevent Immune Overload

A major factor in overactive immune responses is the overproduction of inflammatory cytokines—chemical messengers that signal immune cells to attack threats. When cytokine levels become unbalanced, they can trigger excessive inflammation, leading to tissue damage and worsening symptoms in autoimmune conditions.

DMSO helps regulate this process by:

- **Reducing excessive cytokine activity:** DMSO blocks pro-inflammatory molecules such as TNF-α, IL-6, and IL-1β, which are heavily involved in chronic inflammation and autoimmune disorders.
- **Enhancing anti-inflammatory pathways:** While it suppresses harmful inflammation, DMSO also supports beneficial immune signals, allowing the body to maintain a proper defense against infections.
- **Preventing tissue damage:** By keeping inflammatory responses in check, DMSO reduces collateral damage to healthy tissues, helping to protect organs, joints, and nerves from long-term degradation.

This ability to fine-tune cytokine activity makes DMSO an effective tool in preventing and managing immune system dysfunction, particularly in individuals dealing with chronic inflammatory conditions.

Restoring Immune Balance Without Suppressing Natural Defenses

Traditional immunosuppressant medications, such as steroids and biologics, work by shutting down portions of the immune system. While this approach may reduce symptoms, it also makes individuals more vulnerable to infections and other diseases.

DMSO, on the other hand, offers a different approach:

- **It does not weaken immune function:** Instead of completely shutting down immune activity, DMSO helps the body differentiate between real threats and healthy tissues, reducing autoimmune aggression without increasing susceptibility to infections.
- **It supports detoxification:** Many immune system dysfunctions are worsened by toxic overload from heavy metals, environmental chemicals, and pathogens. DMSO aids in cellular detoxification, helping the immune system function more efficiently and accurately.
- **It enhances antioxidant protection:** Oxidative stress is a major trigger for immune dysfunction, as free radicals damage cells and provoke unnecessary immune responses. DMSO neutralizes these free radicals, helping to restore immune balance naturally.

Reducing Autoimmune Flares and Chronic Inflammation

For individuals with autoimmune conditions, flare-ups are a major concern, often triggered by stress, environmental factors, or infections. These flare-ups lead to pain, fatigue, and organ damage, making symptom management a top priority.

DMSO helps prevent autoimmune flares by:

- Calming the nervous system, reducing stress-related immune overactivation.
- Improving cellular oxygenation, supporting energy production and immune resilience.
- Helping regulate gut health, as imbalances in the microbiome often contribute to immune system dysregulation.

By addressing the underlying mechanisms of immune overactivity, DMSO provides a natural and effective way to restore immune balance, allowing individuals to manage chronic conditions without the risks associated with pharmaceutical immunosuppressants.

Managing Autoimmune Conditions Like Lupus and MS

Autoimmune diseases occur when the immune system mistakenly attacks the body's own tissues, leading to chronic inflammation, organ damage, and debilitating symptoms. Conditions such as lupus (systemic lupus erythematosus, SLE) and multiple sclerosis (MS) are among the most challenging autoimmune disorders, as they affect multiple organ systems and have unpredictable flare-ups. Conventional treatments rely on immunosuppressants, corticosteroids, and biologics, which help control symptoms but often come with severe side effects and increased susceptibility to infections.

DMSO has emerged as a natural, science-backed alternative for managing autoimmune diseases by reducing inflammation, modulating immune responses, and protecting tissues from further damage.

Its ability to penetrate deeply into affected areas, deliver essential nutrients, and neutralize free radicals makes it an effective tool for individuals struggling with autoimmune flare-ups and long-term disease progression.

DMSO and Lupus: Controlling Systemic Inflammation

Lupus is a complex autoimmune disease that causes the immune system to attack healthy organs and tissues, resulting in chronic pain, fatigue, skin rashes, and joint inflammation. It can affect the kidneys, heart, lungs, and brain, making it a multi-system disorder that requires ongoing management.

DMSO provides several benefits for individuals with lupus, including:

- **Reducing systemic inflammation:** Lupus is driven by excessive immune activation, leading to widespread tissue damage. DMSO inhibits inflammatory cytokines (TNF-α, IL-6, IL-1β), reducing pain and swelling in the joints, muscles, and organs.
- **Alleviating joint and muscle pain:** Many lupus patients suffer from chronic pain due to inflammation in the joints and connective tissues. DMSO's natural analgesic properties provide targeted pain relief without the need for high-dose pain medications.
- **Protecting the kidneys and organs:** Lupus nephritis, a serious kidney complication of lupus, occurs when immune cells attack the kidneys' filtering system. DMSO's antioxidant and detoxification properties help reduce oxidative stress, protecting kidney function.
- **Enhancing cellular oxygenation:** Fatigue is a hallmark symptom of lupus, often caused by poor circulation and mitochondrial dysfunction. DMSO improves oxygen transport, helping individuals feel more energized and less fatigued.

By targeting inflammation at the root, DMSO helps control lupus symptoms, allowing individuals to manage their condition with fewer pharmaceutical interventions.

DMSO and Multiple Sclerosis: Supporting Nerve Health and Immune Balance

Multiple sclerosis (MS) is an autoimmune disease that attacks the protective myelin sheath around nerve fibers, leading to neurological symptoms such as muscle weakness, numbness, vision problems, and coordination issues. The progressive nature of MS can result in permanent nerve damage, making it critical to find treatments that slow disease progression while preserving nerve function.

DMSO offers several neuroprotective benefits for individuals with MS:

- **Reducing nerve inflammation:** MS symptoms worsen due to chronic inflammation in the brain and spinal cord. DMSO helps reduce this inflammation by inhibiting pro-inflammatory molecules that contribute to nerve damage.
- **Protecting myelin sheaths:** Myelin is the fatty coating around nerve fibers, essential for proper nerve function. DMSO helps prevent oxidative damage to myelin, reducing the risk of progressive nerve degeneration.
- **Improving circulation in the central nervous system:** Poor circulation in the brain and spinal cord can contribute to neurological decline. DMSO enhances blood flow and nutrient delivery, supporting nerve repair and regeneration.

- **Easing muscle spasms and mobility issues:** Many MS patients experience muscle stiffness, spasms, and coordination problems. DMSO relaxes tight muscles and reduces cramping, helping improve mobility and flexibility.

With its ability to reduce inflammation, protect nerve function, and improve circulation, DMSO presents a promising natural therapy for individuals seeking relief from MS symptoms while supporting long-term neurological health.

DMSO as a Holistic Approach to Autoimmune Disease Management

Lupus and MS are complex conditions with no known cure, but managing symptoms and slowing disease progression is possible with the right approach. DMSO provides immune modulation, pain relief, and cellular protection, making it an effective addition to autoimmune treatment strategies. By addressing both inflammation and tissue damage, DMSO helps individuals maintain better quality of life and greater long-term wellness without the harsh side effects of pharmaceutical immunosuppressants.

CHAPTER 16
DMSO FOR THYROID HEALTH

Supporting Hashimoto's and Hypothyroidism with DMSO

The thyroid is a vital gland responsible for regulating metabolism, energy production, and overall hormonal balance. When it becomes dysfunctional, as in conditions like Hashimoto's thyroiditis and hypothyroidism, individuals experience chronic fatigue, weight gain, brain fog, and a weakened immune system. Conventional treatments typically rely on synthetic hormone replacement, but they do not always address the underlying causes of thyroid dysfunction or reduce inflammation in the gland itself.

DMSO offers a natural and effective approach to supporting thyroid health by reducing autoimmune inflammation, improving cellular oxygenation, and enhancing nutrient absorption. With its powerful anti-inflammatory properties and deep tissue penetration, DMSO may help individuals with Hashimoto's and hypothyroidism manage symptoms and promote thyroid healing at the cellular level.

Regulating Autoimmune Inflammation in Hashimoto's

Hashimoto's thyroiditis is an autoimmune condition in which the immune system mistakenly attacks the thyroid gland, leading to chronic inflammation and gradual destruction of thyroid tissue. Over time, this results in low thyroid hormone production (hypothyroidism), causing fatigue, sluggish metabolism, and difficulty regulating body temperature.

DMSO plays a key role in reducing autoimmune-driven thyroid inflammation by:

- **Modulating the immune response:** DMSO helps suppress overactive immune activity, preventing the thyroid from being continuously attacked.
- **Reducing inflammatory cytokines:** Hashimoto's is associated with high levels of pro-inflammatory molecules such as TNF-α and IL-6, which contribute to thyroid tissue damage. DMSO inhibits these cytokines, helping to protect thyroid cells from further destruction.
- **Detoxifying the thyroid gland:** Environmental toxins, heavy metals, and oxidative stress can exacerbate autoimmune thyroid dysfunction. DMSO is known to bind to harmful compounds, facilitating detoxification and reducing thyroid stress.

By addressing inflammation at the root, DMSO may help individuals with Hashimoto's slow disease progression and support thyroid function naturally.

Improving Thyroid Hormone Absorption and Cellular Oxygenation

One of the challenges in hypothyroidism management is ensuring that thyroid hormones are properly absorbed and utilized by cells. Many individuals on thyroid hormone replacement therapy continue to experience symptoms of low thyroid function, despite taking medication.

DMSO enhances thyroid hormone absorption and efficiency by:

- **Improving cellular oxygenation:** Low thyroid function leads to poor oxygen delivery to cells, contributing to fatigue, brain fog, and slow metabolism. DMSO enhances oxygen transport, boosting energy levels and cognitive function.
- **Enhancing nutrient uptake:** The thyroid requires iodine, selenium, and zinc to produce hormones efficiently. DMSO helps carry these essential nutrients into thyroid cells, optimizing hormone synthesis and activity.
- **Reducing oxidative stress:** The thyroid is highly sensitive to oxidative damage, which can impair hormone production. DMSO acts as a potent antioxidant, protecting thyroid cells from free radical damage.

For individuals struggling with persistent hypothyroid symptoms, DMSO provides a novel approach to improving hormone function, increasing energy, and restoring metabolic balance.

Supporting Overall Thyroid Health and Long-Term Function

Thyroid dysfunction is often a lifelong condition, requiring ongoing management and lifestyle adjustments. While DMSO does not replace conventional treatments, it provides a complementary therapy that helps:

- Reduce inflammation in the thyroid gland
- Improve hormone absorption and efficiency
- Enhance metabolic function and energy production
- Support immune regulation and detoxification

By incorporating DMSO into thyroid health strategies, individuals with Hashimoto's and hypothyroidism may experience better symptom control, increased vitality, and improved overall well-being, without relying solely on pharmaceutical interventions.

DMSO and Selenium: A Powerful Anti-Inflammatory Duo

Inflammation is a key driver of thyroid dysfunction, particularly in conditions such as Hashimoto's thyroiditis and hypothyroidism. When the immune system mistakenly attacks the thyroid, chronic inflammation develops, leading to gradual thyroid tissue destruction and impaired hormone production. While conventional treatments focus on hormone replacement therapy, they do not always address the underlying inflammatory triggers that contribute to ongoing thyroid damage.

DMSO and selenium form a powerful anti-inflammatory combination, working synergistically to reduce oxidative stress, regulate immune function, and support thyroid repair. With DMSO's ability to penetrate deep into tissues and selenium's essential role in thyroid hormone metabolism, this duo presents a natural and science-backed approach to promoting thyroid health and reducing inflammation.

The Role of Selenium in Thyroid Function

Selenium is a critical trace mineral necessary for thyroid hormone production and immune balance. The thyroid contains the highest concentration of selenium in the body, and its deficiency has been linked to increased susceptibility to autoimmune thyroid disorders.

Selenium supports thyroid health by:

- **Regulating the immune system:** Selenium helps balance the immune response, preventing the overactive immune attacks seen in Hashimoto's disease.
- **Reducing thyroid inflammation:** This mineral lowers levels of thyroid-damaging antibodies, such as TPO (thyroid peroxidase) antibodies, which are elevated in autoimmune thyroid conditions.
- **Aiding in thyroid hormone conversion:** Selenium is essential for converting inactive T4 (thyroxine) into the active T3 (triiodothyronine) hormone, ensuring that cells receive sufficient thyroid support.
- **Neutralizing oxidative stress:** The thyroid is highly susceptible to oxidative damage, and selenium plays a vital role in detoxifying harmful free radicals that disrupt thyroid function.

A selenium deficiency can lead to persistent inflammation, increased thyroid antibody levels, and impaired hormone metabolism, making its supplementation a crucial part of thyroid healing protocols.

How DMSO Enhances Selenium Absorption and Effectiveness

While selenium provides critical thyroid protection, its effectiveness can be amplified when paired with DMSO. As a potent anti-inflammatory and transport agent, DMSO enhances selenium's bioavailability and cellular penetration, ensuring that the thyroid and surrounding tissues receive optimal benefits.

DMSO enhances selenium's impact by:

- Carrying selenium deep into thyroid tissues, allowing it to act directly on inflamed or damaged cells.
- Improving blood circulation, ensuring that selenium reaches the thyroid in sufficient quantities.
- Reducing inflammatory cytokines, which helps control excessive immune system activation in autoimmune thyroid disorders.
- Enhancing antioxidant protection, preventing oxidative stress that accelerates thyroid dysfunction.

By combining DMSO's deep tissue penetration with selenium's immune-modulating and anti-inflammatory properties, this combination offers a holistic approach to managing thyroid inflammation and improving overall thyroid function.

Supporting Long-Term Thyroid Health

For individuals struggling with chronic thyroid inflammation, Hashimoto's thyroiditis, or sluggish hormone production, DMSO and selenium together provide a natural and targeted solution. This combination not only addresses inflammation at its root but also supports hormone conversion, immune regulation, and thyroid tissue repair, helping individuals restore thyroid balance and overall well-being.

BOOK 9
DMSO FOR NEUROLOGICAL HEALTH

CHAPTER 17
PROTECTING AND HEALING THE NERVOUS SYSTEM

DMSO for Nerve Regeneration and Repair

The nervous system is one of the most delicate and complex structures in the human body, responsible for transmitting signals between the brain, spinal cord, and the rest of the body. When nerves are damaged due to injury, disease, or chronic inflammation, recovery can be slow and, in some cases, incomplete. Many conventional treatments focus on pain relief rather than true nerve regeneration, leaving patients with persistent discomfort, numbness, or loss of function.

DMSO has gained attention for its unique ability to penetrate nerve tissues, reduce inflammation, and promote cellular repair. Unlike traditional therapies that only provide symptomatic relief, DMSO works at a deeper level, helping to regenerate damaged nerves, restore function, and enhance nerve conduction.

Reducing Nerve Inflammation and Oxidative Stress

Nerve damage is often exacerbated by chronic inflammation and oxidative stress, which impair the ability of nerve cells to repair themselves and function properly. This inflammation can be caused by autoimmune disorders, injuries, toxins, or degenerative conditions like neuropathy.

DMSO helps combat inflammatory damage by:

- **Suppressing pro-inflammatory cytokines:** Excessive levels of TNF-α, IL-6, and IL-1β contribute to nerve swelling and dysfunction. DMSO reduces these inflammatory signals, allowing nerves to heal more efficiently.
- **Neutralizing free radicals:** Nerve cells are highly susceptible to oxidative stress, which accelerates damage. DMSO acts as a powerful antioxidant, preventing cellular breakdown and preserving nerve integrity.
- **Reducing nerve hypersensitivity:** Chronic inflammation often leads to hyperactive nerve responses, causing burning pain, tingling, and heightened sensitivity. By calming these responses, DMSO helps reduce neuropathic discomfort.

This ability to protect nerve cells from further deterioration is essential for individuals dealing with chronic nerve pain, neurodegenerative conditions, or post-injury nerve damage.

Enhancing Nerve Regeneration and Myelin Repair

Damaged nerves require both structural repair and functional recovery, particularly in conditions like peripheral neuropathy, multiple sclerosis, and nerve compression syndromes. One of the biggest challenges in nerve healing is the regeneration of myelin, the protective sheath surrounding nerve fibers.

DMSO promotes nerve healing and repair by:

- **Encouraging nerve cell regeneration:** DMSO enhances the activity of Schwann cells and oligodendrocytes, which are responsible for nerve growth and repair.
- **Promoting myelin restoration:** In conditions where myelin is damaged (such as MS), DMSO helps protect and regenerate this essential nerve insulation, improving nerve signal transmission.
- **Increasing blood flow to nerve tissues:** Adequate circulation is critical for delivering nutrients and oxygen to damaged nerves. DMSO improves vascular function, ensuring better nutrient supply to regenerating neurons.

By addressing both nerve cell repair and functional recovery, DMSO offers a holistic approach to nerve regeneration, helping individuals regain strength, sensation, and proper nerve function.

Restoring Nerve Communication and Function

When nerves are damaged, signal transmission between the brain, spinal cord, and muscles is disrupted, leading to weakness, numbness, or loss of coordination. Even after physical recovery, many individuals experience lingering nerve dysfunction that affects their quality of life.

DMSO enhances nerve communication and function by:

- Improving neurotransmitter signaling, allowing nerves to transmit impulses more efficiently.
- Restoring sensory function, reducing numbness and improving tactile sensation.
- Supporting neuromuscular recovery, helping individuals regain muscle strength and coordination.

For individuals suffering from long-term nerve damage, incorporating DMSO into a nerve regeneration strategy may offer a natural and effective way to restore function and reduce chronic symptoms.

Treating Carpal Tunnel, Sciatica, and Chronic Headaches

Nerve-related conditions such as carpal tunnel syndrome, sciatica, and chronic headaches can be debilitating, persistent, and resistant to conventional treatments. These conditions often result from nerve compression, inflammation, or prolonged stress on nerve pathways, leading to pain, numbness, and reduced mobility. While conventional treatments include painkillers, anti-inflammatory drugs, and even surgical interventions, they often provide only temporary relief without addressing the root cause.

DMSO offers a unique and science-backed alternative by reducing inflammation, improving nerve function, and enhancing circulation to affected areas. With its ability to penetrate deeply into tissues,

DMSO works to relieve pressure on nerves, accelerate healing, and prevent chronic nerve damage in individuals suffering from these painful conditions.

Relieving Carpal Tunnel Syndrome with DMSO

Carpal tunnel syndrome (CTS) occurs when the median nerve is compressed within the wrist, leading to pain, tingling, numbness, and weakness in the hand and fingers. It is often caused by repetitive hand movements, inflammation, or swelling of the tendons in the wrist. Over time, if left untreated, CTS can lead to permanent nerve damage and loss of hand function.

DMSO is particularly effective in managing carpal tunnel syndrome because it:

- Reduces inflammation around the median nerve, relieving pressure and easing pain and tingling sensations.
- Improves circulation to the wrist, helping to reduce swelling and enhance healing.
- Enhances nerve function, allowing for better hand mobility and grip strength.
- Prevents scar tissue formation, which can contribute to worsening nerve compression over time.

For individuals who spend long hours typing, performing manual labor, or using repetitive hand motions, incorporating DMSO into their wrist care routine can help prevent the progression of CTS while alleviating existing symptoms.

Managing Sciatica and Lower Back Nerve Pain

Sciatica is a painful condition caused by compression or irritation of the sciatic nerve, which runs from the lower spine down through the legs. This condition often results in shooting pain, numbness, and muscle weakness in the lower back, hips, and legs. Sciatica can be triggered by herniated discs, spinal misalignment, or prolonged sitting and poor posture.

DMSO provides relief from sciatica pain by:

- Reducing inflammation in the lower back and sciatic nerve, easing pressure and discomfort.
- Increasing blood flow to the affected area, speeding up nerve healing and muscle recovery.
- Relaxing tight muscles around the sciatic nerve, preventing further nerve compression and pain.
- Enhancing cellular repair, allowing damaged nerve fibers to regenerate more effectively.

Individuals struggling with chronic sciatic pain often rely on strong pain medications or invasive procedures, but DMSO offers a natural, non-invasive way to target inflammation at the source and support long-term nerve health.

Addressing Chronic Headaches and Migraines

Chronic headaches, including tension headaches and migraines, can stem from nerve inflammation, poor circulation, or muscle tension in the neck and scalp. Many people with chronic migraines experience symptoms such as light sensitivity, nausea, and throbbing pain, often requiring strong painkillers or pharmaceutical treatments.

DMSO is an effective solution for headache relief because it:

- Reduces inflammation in the nerves and blood vessels of the head, alleviating pressure-induced headaches.
- Relaxes tense muscles in the neck and scalp, improving circulation to the brain.
- Acts as a natural pain reliever, blocking pain signals from overactive nerve pathways.
- Enhances oxygen delivery to the brain, reducing fatigue and brain fog associated with chronic migraines.

For individuals suffering from frequent headaches and migraines, DMSO offers a natural approach to pain management, helping to break the cycle of inflammation and nerve sensitivity that leads to recurrent headaches.

By addressing both the symptoms and underlying causes of carpal tunnel syndrome, sciatica, and chronic headaches, DMSO presents a powerful and holistic solution for those seeking long-lasting relief and improved nerve health.

CHAPTER 18

DMSO AND COGNITIVE FUNCTION

Investigating DMSO for Alzheimer's and Dementia Prevention

Cognitive decline is one of the most pressing health concerns in aging populations, with Alzheimer's disease and other forms of dementia affecting millions worldwide. As these conditions progress, individuals experience memory loss, confusion, impaired decision-making, and a decline in overall brain function. Conventional treatments focus on slowing the disease's progression, but there is still no cure for Alzheimer's or most other forms of dementia.

DMSO has emerged as a potential neuroprotective agent, showing promise in reducing brain inflammation, improving circulation, and protecting neurons from oxidative stress. While research is still ongoing, early findings suggest that DMSO may help delay or even prevent cognitive decline, making it an exciting area of exploration for those looking to preserve brain health naturally.

Reducing Neuroinflammation: A Key to Cognitive Protection

Chronic inflammation in the brain, also known as neuroinflammation, plays a critical role in the development of Alzheimer's and dementia. Inflammatory cytokines, oxidative stress, and the buildup of toxic proteins such as beta-amyloid plaques all contribute to brain cell damage and loss of cognitive function.

DMSO helps combat neuroinflammation by:

- **Suppressing inflammatory cytokines:** High levels of TNF-α, IL-6, and IL-1β are linked to Alzheimer's disease. DMSO reduces these inflammatory molecules, lowering brain inflammation.
- **Neutralizing oxidative stress:** The brain is highly susceptible to oxidative damage, which accelerates neuron degeneration. DMSO is a potent antioxidant, protecting brain cells from free radical damage.
- **Reducing brain swelling and edema:** In conditions like vascular dementia, fluid buildup in the brain can worsen symptoms. DMSO's anti-edema properties help reduce brain swelling and improve cellular function.

By addressing one of the root causes of cognitive decline, DMSO provides a natural, non-toxic approach to supporting long-term brain health.

Improving Blood Flow and Oxygenation to the Brain

One of the hallmarks of dementia is reduced blood circulation to the brain, leading to oxygen deprivation and the gradual loss of neurons. Over time, this contributes to memory impairment, difficulty concentrating, and cognitive fatigue.

DMSO enhances cerebral circulation by:

- Dilating blood vessels, allowing for better oxygen delivery to brain tissues.
- Improving cellular energy production, ensuring that neurons have the resources they need to function efficiently.
- Removing metabolic waste, helping clear toxins that contribute to brain degeneration.

By promoting better circulation and oxygenation, DMSO helps keep neurons active and healthy, reducing the risk of age-related cognitive decline.

Protecting Neurons from Amyloid Plaques and Tau Tangles

In Alzheimer's disease, abnormal proteins called beta-amyloid plaques and tau tangles accumulate in the brain, disrupting communication between neurons and ultimately leading to cell death. Preventing or slowing the formation of these toxic proteins is a major goal in Alzheimer's research.

DMSO may help in this area by:

- **Breaking down protein aggregates:** Early studies suggest that DMSO may help dissolve beta-amyloid plaques, reducing their toxic impact on neurons.
- **Preventing protein misfolding:** Tau proteins become harmful when they misfold and form tangles inside neurons. DMSO helps maintain proper protein structure, preventing the formation of these destructive tangles.
- Enhancing detoxification of harmful compounds, reducing the accumulation of waste products that contribute to brain deterioration.

By protecting brain cells from toxic protein buildup, DMSO offers a promising pathway for slowing the progression of Alzheimer's and related neurodegenerative diseases.

A Natural Approach to Preserving Cognitive Function

For those looking to maintain mental clarity, prevent memory loss, and support long-term brain health, DMSO presents a compelling option. By reducing inflammation, improving circulation, and protecting neurons, it has the potential to delay or even prevent cognitive decline, offering hope to individuals at risk for Alzheimer's and other forms of dementia.

Enhancing Brain Circulation and Reducing Neuroinflammation

The brain relies on optimal circulation and minimal inflammation to function at its highest capacity. When blood flow is restricted, or inflammation becomes chronic, cognitive function suffers, leading to memory loss, brain fog, mental fatigue, and an increased risk of neurodegenerative diseases. Conditions such as Alzheimer's disease, vascular dementia, and cognitive decline are closely linked to poor circulation and excessive neuroinflammation, making these factors critical targets for brain health interventions.

DMSO offers a natural and science-backed approach to improving brain circulation and reducing inflammation, allowing neurons to receive adequate oxygen, essential nutrients, and protection from oxidative damage. By enhancing vascular function and modulating inflammatory responses, DMSO provides a powerful tool for individuals seeking to preserve cognitive function, boost mental clarity, and reduce the risk of neurological disorders.

Improving Blood Flow to the Brain

The brain is a highly energy-demanding organ, requiring constant oxygen and nutrient delivery to function properly. Any disruption in circulation—whether due to aging, vascular issues, or lifestyle factors—can lead to cognitive impairment, reduced mental sharpness, and an increased susceptibility to neurodegenerative diseases.

DMSO enhances cerebral circulation by:

- Dilating blood vessels, allowing for greater oxygen and nutrient delivery to the brain.
- Reducing blood viscosity, improving the flow of blood through capillaries and small vessels.
- Supporting microvascular integrity, preventing capillary damage that can contribute to brain aging and memory decline.
- Increasing oxygen diffusion in brain tissues, optimizing neuronal metabolism and mental clarity.

By boosting blood circulation to the brain, DMSO ensures that neurons receive the necessary energy to function efficiently, helping individuals maintain focus, process information faster, and reduce cognitive fatigue.

Reducing Neuroinflammation and Protecting Brain Cells

Chronic inflammation is a leading cause of cognitive dysfunction, contributing to neuronal damage, impaired signaling, and the buildup of toxic proteins associated with Alzheimer's and other neurodegenerative diseases. The brain has its own immune cells, known as microglia, which regulate inflammation. However, when overactivated, these cells produce excess inflammatory cytokines, leading to chronic neuroinflammation and accelerated brain aging.

DMSO combats neuroinflammation by:

- Regulating microglial activity, preventing excessive immune responses that damage brain tissue.
- Suppressing inflammatory cytokines such as TNF-α, IL-6, and IL-1β, which are linked to cognitive decline and neurodegenerative diseases.

- Neutralizing oxidative stress, which contributes to brain cell death and impaired neurotransmission.
- Protecting the blood-brain barrier, preventing toxins and inflammatory compounds from entering the brain.

By reducing chronic inflammation in the brain, DMSO helps protect neuronal health, enhances cognitive performance, and lowers the risk of age-related brain disorders.

Enhancing Cognitive Function Through Cellular Detoxification

Over time, waste products and metabolic byproducts accumulate in brain tissues, impairing cognitive function and contributing to neurodegenerative conditions. Efficient detoxification is essential for maintaining sharp mental function and preventing brain fog and memory loss.

DMSO enhances cellular detoxification by:

- Flushing out metabolic waste, preventing the buildup of toxins that damage neurons.
- Facilitating the removal of heavy metals and environmental toxins, which are known to contribute to neurological disorders.
- Improving mitochondrial efficiency, ensuring that brain cells have enough energy to function properly.

By supporting brain detoxification and mitochondrial health, DMSO promotes clear thinking, faster recall, and better long-term memory retention.

A Holistic Approach to Brain Health

For individuals looking to maintain cognitive vitality, prevent neurodegenerative diseases, and enhance mental performance, DMSO provides a multi-faceted approach. By boosting circulation, reducing inflammation, and supporting detoxification, it helps optimize brain function naturally, preserving mental clarity and cognitive longevity.

BOOK 10
DMSO FOR DETOX AND HEAVY METAL REMOVAL

CHAPTER 19
DMSO AS A DETOXIFYING AGENT

How DMSO Binds to and Eliminates Heavy Metals

Heavy metal toxicity is an underestimated health threat that can lead to chronic fatigue, cognitive dysfunction, immune suppression, and organ damage. Exposure to mercury, lead, arsenic, aluminum, and cadmium comes from various sources, including industrial pollution, contaminated water, dental fillings, and certain medications. Over time, these toxic metals accumulate in tissues, causing oxidative stress, inflammation, and cellular dysfunction.

Detoxifying the body from these metals is crucial for long-term health, but many conventional detox protocols can be harsh, ineffective, or incomplete. DMSO stands out as a powerful natural detoxifier, capable of binding to heavy metals, breaking them down, and safely eliminating them from the body. Its deep tissue penetration, solvent properties, and ability to cross biological membranes make it uniquely effective in removing toxic accumulations from organs, tissues, and even the brain.

Binding to Heavy Metals at the Cellular Level

One of DMSO's most remarkable properties is its ability to chelate (bind) heavy metals and escort them out of the body. Unlike many other detox agents that work only in the bloodstream, DMSO has the ability to penetrate deep into tissues, where heavy metals accumulate over time.

DMSO binds to heavy metal ions through a process called complexation, forming a soluble, non-toxic compound that can be safely excreted. This allows the body to:

- Mobilize stored heavy metals from tissues, including the brain, liver, and kidneys.
- Reduce metal-induced oxidative stress, preventing further damage to cells.
- Break down metal deposits that contribute to chronic inflammation and immune dysfunction.

By targeting both circulating and tissue-bound heavy metals, DMSO ensures a more comprehensive detoxification process than many conventional methods.

Transporting Heavy Metals Out of the Body

Once DMSO has bound to heavy metals, it facilitates their removal through the body's natural detox pathways. Unlike some chelating agents that rely solely on renal (kidney) excretion, DMSO allows for multiple routes of elimination, ensuring that toxins are efficiently removed.

DMSO promotes heavy metal excretion through:

- **Urine:** Once bound to DMSO, metal complexes are filtered through the kidneys and eliminated via urine, reducing the toxic burden on the body.
- **Sweat:** Due to its skin-penetrating abilities, DMSO allows for some toxins to exit through sweat glands, supporting an additional detoxification route.
- **Lymphatic drainage:** DMSO improves circulatory and lymphatic flow, helping the body clear toxins stored in deep tissues.

By supporting multiple detoxification pathways, DMSO helps prevent metal redistribution, a common issue with less effective chelators that may release metals without properly removing them.

Protecting Cells from Heavy Metal Damage

Heavy metal exposure does not only accumulate toxins in the body—it also generates oxidative stress, which leads to cellular damage, DNA mutations, and chronic inflammation. DMSO not only binds to heavy metals but also protects cells from their harmful effects, preventing long-term damage.

DMSO combats heavy metal toxicity by:

- Neutralizing free radicals, reducing oxidative stress and preventing tissue degradation.
- Stabilizing cell membranes, protecting them from damage caused by metal toxicity.
- Restoring mitochondrial function, which is often impaired by mercury and aluminum toxicity.

By addressing both the presence of heavy metals and the damage they cause, DMSO offers a comprehensive and highly effective detoxification strategy, supporting optimal health and cellular longevity.

Supporting Liver and Kidney Function During Detox

The liver and kidneys are the body's primary detoxification organs, responsible for filtering out toxins, metabolizing waste, and maintaining overall health. When heavy metals, environmental pollutants, and metabolic byproducts accumulate in the body, these organs must work harder to eliminate them. Over time, toxic overload can impair liver and kidney function, leading to fatigue, inflammation, and weakened immunity.

DMSO plays a unique role in detoxification by not only binding to toxins and transporting them out of the body but also supporting liver and kidney function during the process. Unlike some harsh detox protocols that may strain these organs, DMSO enhances their ability to process and eliminate toxins efficiently, preventing detox-related side effects such as headaches, nausea, and fatigue.

Reducing Liver Burden and Enhancing Detox Pathways

The liver is the body's main detox organ, responsible for breaking down harmful substances, neutralizing free radicals, and excreting waste through bile and urine. However, exposure to toxins, medications, and heavy metals can lead to liver congestion and inflammation, making detoxification less effective.

DMSO supports liver function by:

- Enhancing liver cell regeneration, helping hepatocytes (liver cells) repair from toxin-induced damage.
- Improving bile flow, allowing the liver to efficiently excrete heavy metals and fat-soluble toxins.
- Neutralizing oxidative stress, which can lead to inflammation and liver dysfunction.
- Reducing fibrosis risk, preventing the buildup of scar tissue in the liver caused by prolonged toxin exposure.

By protecting the liver and enhancing its detox capabilities, DMSO ensures that toxins are metabolized more efficiently, reducing the risk of toxin recirculation in the body.

Supporting Kidney Function for Efficient Toxin Elimination

The kidneys play a critical role in filtering the blood, removing waste products, and balancing electrolytes. During detoxification, toxins mobilized from tissues must be processed through the kidneys, increasing their workload. If the kidneys are overwhelmed or sluggish, toxin elimination slows down, leading to fluid retention, inflammation, and toxin buildup in the bloodstream.

DMSO enhances kidney function by:

- Increasing renal blood flow, ensuring toxins are effectively filtered and eliminated through urine.
- Reducing oxidative damage in kidney tissues, protecting nephrons (kidney cells) from heavy metal toxicity.
- Promoting diuresis (urine production), facilitating faster toxin clearance.
- Preventing kidney stone formation, by reducing calcium oxalate and uric acid deposits that can accumulate during detox.

By supporting kidney filtration and toxin elimination, DMSO ensures that waste products are efficiently removed, preventing detox symptoms such as bloating, fatigue, and brain fog.

Minimizing Detox Reactions and Enhancing Cellular Protection

During detoxification, toxins are released from tissues and enter circulation, which can sometimes lead to temporary side effects such as headaches, fatigue, or nausea. This is known as a detox reaction, and it occurs when the body struggles to process and eliminate toxins quickly enough.

DMSO helps minimize detox reactions by:

- Reducing inflammation caused by circulating toxins, easing detox-related discomfort.
- Enhancing cellular protection, preventing toxins from damaging healthy cells during elimination.
- Improving mitochondrial function, ensuring that cells have enough energy to process toxins effectively.

By protecting liver and kidney function while accelerating toxin clearance, DMSO offers a powerful and efficient way to detox without overburdening the body's natural filtration systems.

CHAPTER 20
ADVANCED DETOX PROTOCOLS WITH DMSO

Combining DMSO with Activated Charcoal and Vitamin C

Detoxification is a multi-step process that involves binding, neutralizing, and eliminating toxins from the body. While DMSO is a powerful detoxifying agent on its own, combining it with activated charcoal and vitamin C enhances its effectiveness, ensuring that toxins are not only mobilized but also safely removed from the body.

Activated charcoal acts as a binding agent, capturing toxins and preventing them from being reabsorbed, while vitamin C provides antioxidant protection and supports liver function. This strategic combination allows for a more efficient, safer detox process, minimizing side effects and optimizing cellular health.

The Role of DMSO in Detoxification

DMSO plays a unique role in detox protocols, as it is one of the few natural compounds capable of penetrating deep into tissues and mobilizing toxins stored in fat, organs, and cells. Unlike many detox agents that only target circulating toxins, DMSO is able to extract deeply embedded heavy metals, pesticides, and other pollutants, making it a powerful first step in a detox regimen.

DMSO's detoxifying effects include:

- Binding to heavy metals and toxins, allowing for easier elimination.
- Reducing inflammation, preventing oxidative damage during detox.
- Enhancing nutrient absorption, ensuring that detox-supporting compounds like vitamin C reach the cells more efficiently.
- Supporting cellular repair, helping the body heal from toxin-induced damage.

However, mobilizing toxins is only half the battle—without proper elimination, they can be reabsorbed into the bloodstream, leading to detox reactions such as fatigue, nausea, and headaches. This is where activated charcoal and vitamin C become essential.

Activated Charcoal: Capturing and Eliminating Toxins

Once toxins are mobilized by DMSO, activated charcoal helps bind to them in the digestive tract, preventing them from re-entering circulation and ensuring that they are safely removed through the bowels.

Activated charcoal enhances detox by:

- Adsorbing toxins, trapping heavy metals, pesticides, and environmental pollutants.
- Preventing toxin recirculation, reducing detox-related symptoms.
- Supporting digestive health, aiding in gut microbiome balance by absorbing harmful substances.

Because activated charcoal is highly porous, it works like a magnet for toxins, ensuring that they are fully excreted from the body without lingering effects or reabsorption.

Vitamin C: Antioxidant Protection and Liver Support

Detoxification can place temporary stress on the body, leading to increased oxidative damage as toxins are broken down and processed. Vitamin C plays a critical role in neutralizing free radicals, ensuring that detoxification happens without harming healthy cells.

Vitamin C supports detox by:

- Enhancing liver enzyme function, allowing toxins to be processed efficiently.
- Neutralizing free radicals, protecting cells from detox-related oxidative stress.
- Boosting the immune system, helping the body recover from toxin exposure.
- Supporting collagen production, which aids in tissue repair after detox.

By working together, DMSO, activated charcoal, and vitamin C form a powerful trio, ensuring that toxins are mobilized, bound, and safely eliminated, while also protecting the body from the stress of detoxification.

Safely Implementing a Long-Term Detox Plan

Detoxification is not just a one-time event but a continuous process that allows the body to eliminate toxins, maintain optimal function, and prevent chronic disease. While short-term detox protocols can provide immediate relief from toxic overload, a long-term detox plan ensures that the body remains in a state of balance, reducing inflammation and enhancing cellular health.

DMSO is a powerful detoxifier, but its long-term use must be approached strategically and safely. Detoxing too aggressively or without proper support for the liver, kidneys, and immune system can lead to unwanted side effects, including fatigue, headaches, and digestive discomfort. Implementing a structured detox plan that gradually integrates DMSO along with dietary support, hydration, and targeted supplementation allows for sustainable toxin removal without overburdening the body.

Balancing Detoxification with Cellular Support

When implementing a long-term detox plan, the key is to support detox pathways while simultaneously nourishing the body. Detoxification happens in three phases:

- **Phase 1:** Toxin Mobilization: Stored toxins in fat, organs, and tissues are released into circulation.
- **Phase 2:** Toxin Neutralization: The liver processes and converts toxins into forms that can be excreted.
- **Phase 3:** Toxin Elimination: The kidneys, bowels, and sweat glands work to remove toxins from the body.

A safe detox plan ensures that each of these phases is supported so that toxins do not recirculate and cause harm.

DMSO is highly effective at mobilizing toxins, but without proper elimination support, reabsorbed toxins can lead to detox reactions. This is why hydration, liver support, and mineral replenishment must be prioritized throughout the process.

Preventing Detox Overload and Managing Symptoms

As the body eliminates toxins, it may go through temporary adjustment periods, often referred to as detox symptoms or healing crises. These may include:

- **Headaches and brain fog:** A sign that toxins are being mobilized but need to be flushed out.
- **Fatigue and muscle aches:** The result of toxin circulation and temporary mineral depletion.
- **Digestive discomfort:** The liver and gut work hard to process and eliminate toxic substances.

To minimize detox reactions and prevent overwhelming the system, it's essential to:

- Start with a low and slow approach, gradually increasing detox intensity over time.
- Support liver function with nutrients like milk thistle, glutathione, and vitamin C.
- Stay hydrated to assist the kidneys in flushing out toxins.
- Ensure regular bowel movements to prevent toxin reabsorption in the gut.
- Incorporate gentle movement to stimulate lymphatic drainage and circulation.

By balancing detoxification with proper elimination support, the body can remove toxins efficiently without unnecessary stress.

Integrating Detox into Daily Life

A long-term detox plan should be sustainable and adaptable, allowing individuals to incorporate detox strategies into their daily routines. This includes:

- Eating a nutrient-dense diet rich in antioxidants and anti-inflammatory foods.
- Minimizing toxin exposure by reducing processed foods, plastics, and environmental pollutants.
- Using periodic detox phases to clear accumulated toxins while allowing for recovery periods.

- Maintaining gut health to ensure proper digestion and toxin elimination.

By following a structured long-term detox plan, the body remains in a state of optimal function, allowing for ongoing cellular repair, improved energy levels, and long-term vitality.

…

BOOK 11
DMSO IN CANCER THERAPY SUPPORT

CHAPTER 21

HOW DMSO ASSISTS CANCER TREATMENT

Enhancing Chemotherapy Absorption While Reducing Side Effects

Chemotherapy is a powerful but aggressive cancer treatment that targets rapidly dividing cells, aiming to eliminate tumors and prevent metastasis. However, the systemic toxicity of chemotherapy often leads to significant side effects, including nausea, fatigue, weakened immunity, and organ stress. While it is an essential component of conventional cancer treatment, improving the efficiency of drug absorption while minimizing damage to healthy tissues remains a critical goal in oncology.

DMSO has gained attention as a potential adjunct therapy to chemotherapy due to its unique ability to enhance drug delivery, protect healthy cells, and reduce treatment-related toxicity. By acting as a penetration enhancer, DMSO improves chemotherapy absorption at the cellular level, ensuring that cancer-fighting drugs reach tumors more efficiently while sparing non-cancerous tissues.

Improving Chemotherapy Drug Penetration

One of the primary challenges of chemotherapy is drug resistance and uneven drug distribution. Many chemotherapy agents struggle to penetrate deep into tumor tissues, limiting their effectiveness. Additionally, cancer cells can develop mechanisms to expel drugs, reducing their potency over time.

DMSO enhances chemotherapy drug absorption by:

- Increasing membrane permeability, allowing chemotherapeutic agents to enter cells more efficiently.
- Bypassing cellular resistance mechanisms, ensuring that drugs are not rejected before exerting their effects.
- Targeting cancer cells more precisely, reducing the need for excessive dosages.

This enhanced absorption allows chemotherapy to be more effective at lower doses, potentially reducing the need for high-intensity treatments that cause severe side effects.

Protecting Healthy Cells from Chemotherapy-Induced Damage

A major drawback of chemotherapy is its non-selective nature, meaning it targets both cancerous and healthy cells. This widespread cellular damage is what leads to common chemotherapy side effects, such as immune suppression, digestive distress, and neuropathy.

DMSO helps shield healthy cells by:

- Acting as an antioxidant, neutralizing chemotherapy-induced free radicals that cause DNA damage.
- Reducing inflammation, preventing excessive tissue damage and preserving organ function.
- Enhancing cellular repair mechanisms, allowing healthy tissues to recover faster after chemotherapy exposure.

By minimizing collateral damage, DMSO can potentially make chemotherapy more tolerable, improving quality of life for patients undergoing treatment.

Reducing Chemotherapy Side Effects and Toxicity

The accumulation of chemotherapy-related toxins in the body contributes to severe side effects, often requiring dose adjustments or treatment interruptions. DMSO facilitates toxin clearance and helps mitigate common chemotherapy-related symptoms.

DMSO supports detoxification by:

- Enhancing liver function, assisting in the breakdown and removal of chemotherapy metabolites.
- Supporting kidney filtration, preventing toxic buildup that can lead to renal stress and electrolyte imbalances.
- Reducing oxidative stress, preventing long-term tissue damage caused by chemotherapy-induced toxicity.

By improving detoxification pathways, DMSO allows patients to recover more quickly between treatment cycles, reducing the burden on the body's elimination systems.

Aiding in Drug Transport Across the Blood-Brain Barrier

For cancers affecting the brain and nervous system, chemotherapy is often less effective due to the protective nature of the blood-brain barrier (BBB), which limits the entry of large molecules, including many chemotherapeutic agents.

DMSO is known for its ability to cross the BBB, making it a potential carrier for chemotherapy drugs targeting brain tumors. By improving drug delivery to the central nervous system, DMSO may enhance the efficacy of treatments for glioblastoma, metastatic brain cancer, and other neurological malignancies.

By optimizing drug absorption, reducing toxicity, and improving cellular resilience, DMSO presents a compelling tool in integrative cancer treatment, potentially enhancing the effectiveness and tolerability of chemotherapy protocols.

DMSO and Oxygen Therapy: Improving Cellular Oxygenation

Oxygen is essential for cellular metabolism, energy production, and overall health. However, in many chronic conditions, including cancer, neurodegenerative diseases, and cardiovascular disorders, oxygen delivery to tissues becomes compromised. Hypoxia (low oxygen levels) can create an environment where damaged cells thrive, particularly in cancer, where tumors often develop in oxygen-deficient regions.

DMSO has gained attention for its ability to enhance oxygen transport and improve cellular oxygenation. When combined with oxygen therapy, DMSO may increase oxygen uptake in tissues, reduce inflammation, and support mitochondrial function, making it a valuable tool for individuals seeking to restore cellular energy and combat disease.

How DMSO Enhances Oxygen Absorption

One of DMSO's most unique properties is its high solubility in water and fat, allowing it to carry molecules, including oxygen, deep into tissues. This characteristic makes it particularly useful in oxygen-deprived environments, such as those found in damaged, inflamed, or cancerous tissues.

DMSO enhances oxygen absorption by:

- Transporting oxygen molecules across cell membranes, ensuring that tissues receive adequate oxygen supply.
- Improving microcirculation, allowing oxygen-rich blood to reach hypoxic (low-oxygen) areas more efficiently.
- Reducing oxidative stress, preventing cellular damage caused by low oxygen levels and free radical accumulation.
- Enhancing mitochondrial function, optimizing ATP (energy) production within cells.

By increasing oxygen availability, DMSO may support cell repair, immune function, and overall vitality, making it a promising adjunct to oxygen-based therapies.

DMSO and Hyperbaric Oxygen Therapy (HBOT)

Hyperbaric Oxygen Therapy (HBOT) is a treatment that involves breathing pure oxygen in a pressurized chamber, allowing for greater oxygen absorption in the body. This therapy is used for wound healing, neurological recovery, and immune support, but its effectiveness can be further enhanced with DMSO.

DMSO complements HBOT by:

- Increasing tissue permeability, allowing oxygen to penetrate deep into damaged areas.
- Reducing inflammation and swelling, improving circulation and enhancing oxygen delivery.
- Detoxifying the body, removing metabolic waste that may interfere with oxygen uptake.

By working together, DMSO and HBOT provide a synergistic effect, optimizing oxygen absorption at the cellular level and promoting faster recovery from injury or illness.

DMSO and Ozone Therapy: A Potent Detoxification Combination

Ozone therapy is another oxygen-based treatment that delivers O3 (ozone) molecules into the bloodstream to combat chronic infections, inflammation, and oxidative stress. Like HBOT, ozone therapy can benefit from the transport-enhancing effects of DMSO.

DMSO amplifies ozone therapy by:

- Enhancing oxygen diffusion in tissues, making ozone therapy more effective at increasing cellular oxygenation.
- Neutralizing toxic byproducts, reducing oxidative damage from reactive oxygen species (ROS).
- Stimulating detox pathways, ensuring that oxygen metabolism byproducts are efficiently removed.

When combined, DMSO and oxygen therapies create a powerful synergy, promoting tissue regeneration, immune function, and metabolic balance, offering potential benefits for a wide range of chronic health conditions.

CHAPTER 22
ALTERNATIVE CANCER PROTOCOLS WITH DMSO

Combining DMSO with High-Dose Vitamin C and Herbal Treatments

In the realm of alternative cancer therapies, the combination of DMSO, high-dose vitamin C, and herbal treatments has gained attention for its synergistic effects on immune support, oxidative stress reduction, and cellular detoxification. While conventional treatments like chemotherapy and radiation focus on directly eliminating cancer cells, this alternative approach aims to enhance the body's natural defenses, improve nutrient absorption, and promote overall healing.

DMSO plays a critical role in this protocol by enhancing the delivery of vitamin C and herbal compounds deep into tissues, ensuring that their therapeutic properties reach the cellular level where they can exert their maximum benefits. By combining these natural compounds, individuals seeking complementary or integrative cancer support may experience improved well-being, reduced side effects, and enhanced recovery.

The Role of DMSO in Enhancing Vitamin C Absorption

Vitamin C is one of the most well-known antioxidants and immune boosters, with research suggesting that high doses may help slow cancer progression, reduce inflammation, and support cellular repair. However, one of the challenges with high-dose vitamin C therapy is bioavailability—only a fraction of the vitamin C taken orally reaches the bloodstream due to digestive limitations and rapid excretion.

DMSO improves vitamin C absorption by:

- Acting as a carrier molecule, transporting vitamin C directly into cells, bypassing digestion.
- Allowing deeper tissue penetration, ensuring that high-dose vitamin C reaches tumors and inflamed areas.
- Enhancing antioxidant activity, reducing oxidative stress and neutralizing free radicals more effectively.
- Prolonging vitamin C retention in the body, ensuring sustained therapeutic benefits.

By increasing cellular uptake of vitamin C, DMSO enhances its immune-boosting, anti-inflammatory, and detoxifying effects, making it a powerful addition to high-dose vitamin C therapy.

Harnessing the Power of Herbal Treatments

Herbs have been used for centuries to support immune function, detoxify the body, and promote cellular health. In cancer support protocols, certain anti-inflammatory, adaptogenic, and immune-modulating herbs have shown potential in reducing tumor growth, enhancing detox pathways, and improving overall vitality.

DMSO enhances the effectiveness of herbal treatments by:

- Transporting active compounds into cells, maximizing their absorption.
- Reducing systemic inflammation, creating an environment less favorable for cancer progression.
- Supporting detoxification, ensuring that metabolic waste and toxins from cell die-off are effectively removed.

Common herbs used in DMSO-assisted cancer protocols include:

- **Turmeric (Curcumin):** A powerful anti-inflammatory that may inhibit cancer cell proliferation.
- **Milk Thistle:** Supports liver detoxification, helping the body process toxins more efficiently.
- **Essiac Tea (Burdock Root, Sheep Sorrel, Slippery Elm, Rhubarb Root):** Traditionally used to support the immune system and aid in cancer recovery.
- **Pau d'Arco:** Known for its antifungal and antimicrobial properties, helping the body combat infections and inflammation.

By combining DMSO, vitamin C, and targeted herbal therapies, this approach supports immune function, reduces oxidative stress, and enhances cellular detoxification, creating a comprehensive strategy for holistic cancer support.

Success Stories of DMSO in Cancer Support

Over the years, patients, alternative medicine practitioners, and researchers have explored DMSO as a supportive therapy in cancer treatment. While DMSO is not a conventional cancer cure, its unique properties in reducing inflammation, enhancing drug absorption, and supporting detoxification have made it an attractive option for individuals seeking complementary approaches. Across the world, there are numerous accounts of patients who have incorporated DMSO into their protocols and experienced remarkable improvements in pain management, chemotherapy tolerance, and overall well-being.

Regaining Strength and Reducing Chemotherapy Side Effects

One of the most common challenges for cancer patients undergoing chemotherapy or radiation therapy is the severe side effects—nausea, fatigue, pain, and immune suppression. Some individuals have reported that incorporating DMSO alongside their prescribed treatments has helped them tolerate the process with fewer side effects and faster recovery times.

- **Case Example:** A middle-aged woman undergoing treatment for breast cancer struggled with crippling fatigue and nausea after each chemotherapy session. After working with an integrative doctor, she began applying DMSO topically alongside high-dose vitamin C therapy. Within a few weeks, she noticed a significant reduction in nausea, improved energy levels, and less discomfort following chemotherapy sessions.

Many similar reports indicate that DMSO's ability to carry nutrients into cells enhances the effectiveness of antioxidant therapy, helping the body counteract the oxidative damage caused by chemotherapy drugs.

Pain Reduction and Improved Quality of Life

For cancer patients, chronic pain—whether from tumors pressing on nerves, surgical interventions, or the effects of radiation—can be debilitating. Some individuals have turned to DMSO for its natural analgesic and anti-inflammatory properties, allowing them to manage pain without relying solely on opioids or heavy medications.

- **Case Example:** A man diagnosed with pancreatic cancer suffered from severe abdominal pain that limited his ability to eat and sleep. Seeking relief, he began using DMSO in combination with herbal anti-inflammatories, such as turmeric and boswellia. Over time, he experienced noticeable pain reduction, which enabled him to eat better, sleep more comfortably, and engage in light physical activity again.

While pain management varies from patient to patient, reports suggest that DMSO's ability to penetrate deep into tissues and reduce inflammation makes it a valuable tool for managing discomfort associated with cancer and its treatments.

Hope for Those Who Were Told There Were No Options Left

One of the most compelling aspects of DMSO in cancer support is its use by individuals who have exhausted conventional options and sought alternative methods to maintain their quality of life. While every case is unique, some individuals have shared their experiences of using DMSO in combination with other therapies and seeing improvements in their condition.

- **Case Example:** A retired teacher was diagnosed with advanced prostate cancer and given a poor prognosis. Facing limited conventional options, he began an integrative protocol involving DMSO, ozone therapy, and a nutrient-rich diet. Over time, his energy levels increased, pain decreased, and his tumor markers stabilized, allowing him to continue living actively and engaging with his family.

These accounts do not suggest that DMSO is a stand-alone cancer cure, but they illustrate how DMSO, when combined with other natural or conventional treatments, may improve quality of life, reduce symptoms, and support the body's healing mechanisms.

BOOK 12
DMSO FOR VETERINARY USE

CHAPTER 23
TREATING PETS AND LIVESTOCK WITH DMSO

Arthritis, Inflammation, and Injury Recovery in Animals

Just like humans, animals suffer from arthritis, inflammation, and injuries, especially as they age or engage in high-intensity activities. Dogs, cats, horses, and livestock frequently experience joint stiffness, ligament tears, muscle soreness, and chronic pain, making mobility difficult and reducing their quality of life. Traditional veterinary treatments often include anti-inflammatory drugs, painkillers, and steroid injections, but these come with potential side effects, including liver strain, digestive issues, and dependency.

DMSO has emerged as a natural alternative for managing arthritis, inflammation, and injury recovery in animals, thanks to its powerful anti-inflammatory, pain-relieving, and tissue-healing properties. It is widely used in equine therapy, veterinary medicine, and holistic pet care, providing a safer, drug-free approach to improving mobility and reducing discomfort.

How DMSO Reduces Arthritis and Joint Inflammation in Pets

Arthritis is a progressive condition caused by cartilage degradation, chronic inflammation, and joint stiffness. It is especially common in older dogs, large-breed dogs, racehorses, and senior cats. Traditional treatments often focus on masking pain rather than addressing the underlying inflammation, leading to long-term medication dependency.

DMSO helps alleviate arthritis symptoms by:

- **Reducing joint inflammation:** It penetrates deeply into tissues, reducing swelling and stiffness.
- **Acting as a pain modulator:** It interrupts pain signals, offering long-lasting relief without the side effects of NSAIDs.
- **Improving circulation:** It enhances blood flow to arthritic joints, ensuring nutrient delivery and waste removal.
- **Preventing further joint deterioration:** By reducing oxidative stress, it helps protect cartilage from further breakdown.

Many dog owners and horse trainers have reported increased mobility, reduced limping, and improved activity levels in animals treated with DMSO.

DMSO for Injury Recovery in Working and Sporting Animals

For active and working animals, injuries are common due to overuse, accidents, and strain on muscles, tendons, and ligaments. Horses in racing, jumping, and endurance events often experience tendonitis, ligament injuries, and muscle soreness, while dogs engaged in agility sports or herding may develop joint sprains and soft tissue damage.

DMSO accelerates injury recovery by:

- **Reducing swelling and bruising:** It prevents fluid buildup, minimizing post-injury inflammation.
- **Enhancing tissue repair:** It promotes collagen production, speeding up ligament and tendon healing.
- **Improving flexibility and reducing stiffness:** Helps restore range of motion faster than conventional treatments.

Veterinary professionals and animal caregivers have found that DMSO significantly shortens healing times, allowing horses, dogs, and livestock to return to activity sooner while reducing the need for steroids or prescription pain medications.

Supporting Chronic Pain Conditions and Age-Related Degeneration

As animals age, they become more prone to degenerative conditions like:

- Hip dysplasia (common in large dog breeds)
- Spinal arthritis and nerve compression
- Post-surgical recovery inflammation
- Chronic pain from old injuries

DMSO has been used to support aging animals, offering them a higher quality of life, better mobility, and reduced pain without the risks of long-term drug use. Owners often note increased energy, willingness to move, and overall improvement in their pet's comfort levels after incorporating DMSO into their wellness routine.

Safe Dosages for Dogs, Cats, and Horses

DMSO is widely used in veterinary medicine for its anti-inflammatory, pain-relieving, and healing properties. However, ensuring the correct dosage for each species is crucial for safety and effectiveness. Because DMSO is a potent carrier agent, it quickly absorbs into tissues and can transport other substances with it. This makes it essential to use pure, high-quality DMSO and follow safe dilution and application guidelines for dogs, cats, and horses.

Understanding Proper Dosage and Application

The correct dosage of DMSO depends on several factors, including:

- The size and weight of the animal
- The method of administration (topical, oral, or injection—though veterinary guidance is required for injections)
- The condition being treated (inflammation, arthritis, injury, or post-surgical recovery)
- The animal's tolerance and sensitivity to DMSO

DMSO is typically used in topical applications, but in some veterinary settings, it may be diluted for oral use. However, because of its strong solvent properties, oral administration should only be under the supervision of a veterinarian.

DMSO Dosage for Dogs

Dogs generally tolerate low concentrations of DMSO well, but dosage should be carefully measured to avoid irritation.

- **Topical Use:** A 50% DMSO solution (diluted with distilled water or aloe vera) can be applied to inflamed joints, sore muscles, or injuries.
- **Application Frequency:** No more than twice daily to avoid skin irritation.
- **Oral Use:** Only under veterinary supervision, and usually in very low doses mixed with water.

Dogs may experience garlic-like breath odor after DMSO absorption, which is a normal side effect due to its metabolic breakdown.

DMSO Dosage for Cats: Use with Extreme Caution

Cats are highly sensitive to DMSO because their liver enzymes metabolize substances differently than other animals. Many veterinarians recommend against using DMSO in cats, except under professional supervision.

- **Topical Use:** Only in very low concentrations (10-20%), applied sparingly to affected areas.
- **Avoid Oral Administration:** Cats are particularly sensitive to toxicity, and ingestion should be avoided unless recommended by a veterinarian.

Due to their unique metabolism, cats may develop gastrointestinal upset, excessive salivation, or lethargy if exposed to high concentrations of DMSO.

DMSO Dosage for Horses

Horses are commonly treated with DMSO in veterinary medicine, particularly for joint inflammation, tendon injuries, and swelling.

- **Topical Use:** A 70-90% DMSO solution is often used for horses, as they tolerate higher concentrations than smaller animals.

- **Application Frequency:** 1-2 times per day on affected areas, avoiding overuse to prevent skin irritation.
- **Oral or IV Use:** Only performed by veterinarians for specific conditions, such as neurological swelling or colic-related inflammation.

Because horses have large body mass, they require higher dosages, but careful monitoring is essential to avoid adverse effects.

By following species-specific guidelines, DMSO can be a safe and effective therapy for managing pain, inflammation, and injuries in animals.

CHAPTER 24
ADVANCED VETERINARY APPLICATIONS

DMSO for Equine Performance and Racehorse Recovery

The world of equine sports and racing places immense physical demands on horses. Speed, endurance, and agility are critical, but these high-performance activities often come with strain, injury, and inflammation. Trainers, veterinarians, and horse owners are constantly seeking safe and effective methods to enhance performance, recovery, and overall joint health.

DMSO has become a trusted tool in the equine industry due to its powerful anti-inflammatory, pain-relieving, and tissue-healing properties. Used for both recovery and performance optimization, DMSO allows racehorses to bounce back from injuries, reduce stiffness, and improve mobility, ensuring they remain in top condition.

Enhancing Performance Through Faster Recovery

Equine athletes experience constant muscle exertion, joint impact, and soft tissue strain. Even when not injured, horses can develop microtears in muscles, joint soreness, and lactic acid buildup, all of which can hinder performance and slow recovery times.

DMSO aids performance by:

- Reducing post-exercise inflammation, helping muscles recover more quickly.
- Enhancing circulation, allowing oxygen and nutrients to reach fatigued tissues faster.
- Breaking down lactic acid accumulation, preventing stiffness and soreness after races or training.
- Maintaining joint flexibility, crucial for horses that perform repetitive high-impact movements.

By accelerating muscle repair and reducing inflammation, DMSO supports consistent performance levels, allowing racehorses to train harder without the risk of excessive wear and tear.

Treating Tendon and Ligament Injuries in Racehorses

One of the most common injuries in racehorses and performance horses involves tendon and ligament damage. These injuries are challenging to heal, requiring long rest periods and extensive rehabilitation. DMSO is widely used in equine sports medicine to aid in faster tendon repair, reduce swelling, and restore mobility.

DMSO works by:

- Deeply penetrating soft tissue, reaching affected ligaments and tendons where conventional treatments struggle to be effective.
- Reducing fluid buildup and inflammation, preventing excessive swelling that can delay healing.
- Protecting against oxidative stress, which can degrade tendon fibers and slow recovery.

Horses that receive DMSO applications soon after an injury often show faster improvement, with reduced downtime and fewer complications.

Supporting Joint Health for Long-Term Career Longevity

One of the biggest concerns in racing and competitive equine sports is joint degeneration. Horses subjected to repetitive motion, high-speed impact, and hard track surfaces often develop arthritis, joint inflammation, and cartilage wear at an early age.

DMSO plays a preventative role in joint health by:

- Lubricating joints and reducing stiffness, keeping movement fluid and pain-free.
- Reducing oxidative damage, preserving cartilage integrity for long-term mobility.
- Enhancing absorption of joint-supporting nutrients, improving the effectiveness of supplements like glucosamine and chondroitin.

By incorporating DMSO into post-training care and recovery routines, trainers can extend a horse's athletic career, reduce strain-related injuries, and maintain long-term joint function.

DMSO remains a cornerstone of equine therapy, offering fast-acting relief, accelerated recovery, and improved overall performance for racehorses, show horses, and working equines alike.

Treating Skin Conditions and Infections in Pets

Skin conditions in pets are among the most common reasons for veterinary visits, affecting dogs, cats, and other companion animals. Issues such as hot spots, fungal infections, bacterial dermatitis, and allergic reactions can cause discomfort, excessive itching, hair loss, and even secondary infections if left untreated. While traditional treatments like antibiotics, corticosteroids, and antifungal medications can be effective, they often come with side effects, long-term dependency, or reduced efficacy over time.

DMSO has gained recognition in veterinary care for its powerful anti-inflammatory, antimicrobial, and wound-healing properties. By penetrating deep into tissues, it helps reduce inflammation, accelerate healing, and improve medication absorption, making it a valuable tool for managing various skin conditions in pets.

DMSO for Bacterial and Fungal Skin Infections

Bacterial and fungal infections are common in pets, especially in humid environments or among animals with weakened immune systems. Conditions like staphylococcal infections (staph), ringworm, and yeast overgrowth can cause redness, scaling, crusty patches, and persistent itching.

DMSO helps fight skin infections by:

- Acting as a natural antimicrobial agent, inhibiting bacterial and fungal growth.
- Penetrating deep into infected tissues, reaching microorganisms that topical treatments may not fully eradicate.
- Reducing inflammation and swelling, easing discomfort and promoting faster healing.
- Enhancing the effects of antifungal and antibacterial treatments, ensuring better absorption into affected areas.

When applied correctly and in the appropriate concentration, DMSO can help resolve persistent skin infections without the need for long-term pharmaceutical reliance.

Managing Allergic Reactions and Hot Spots

Many pets suffer from allergic skin conditions, often caused by environmental allergens, food sensitivities, or flea bites. Allergic reactions lead to intense itching, hair loss, and self-inflicted wounds, creating a vicious cycle of scratching and irritation.

DMSO plays a key role in soothing allergic skin reactions by:

- Reducing histamine release, minimizing allergic flare-ups.
- Calming inflamed and irritated skin, preventing pets from excessive scratching.
- Accelerating tissue repair, helping wounds from self-inflicted scratching heal faster.

Hot spots—moist, inflamed skin lesions caused by excessive licking, scratching, or bacterial infections—can spread rapidly if untreated. DMSO's quick absorption and anti-inflammatory properties help dry out and heal hot spots, providing relief without the side effects of steroids.

Wound Healing and Post-Surgical Recovery

DMSO is widely used in veterinary wound management, particularly for minor cuts, abrasions, burns, and post-surgical recovery. By increasing blood circulation and oxygenation to injured tissues, DMSO supports:

- Faster wound closure, reducing scarring.
- Lower risk of infection, thanks to its natural antiseptic properties.
- Pain relief, ensuring greater comfort for the animal during healing.

By incorporating DMSO into skin care treatments for pets, owners and veterinarians can help manage chronic skin conditions, speed up healing, and improve overall skin health, making it an invaluable addition to holistic pet care regimens.

BOOK 13
HIGH-DOSE DMSO THERAPY AND CLINICAL APPLICATIONS

CHAPTER 25
ADVANCED CLINICAL USES OF DMSO

DMSO Therapy for Lyme Disease and Chronic Conditions

Lyme disease and other chronic inflammatory conditions pose a significant challenge for both patients and healthcare providers. These illnesses often lead to persistent fatigue, joint pain, neurological symptoms, and systemic inflammation, making daily life difficult. Many individuals struggling with chronic Lyme disease, fibromyalgia, or autoimmune disorders find little relief with conventional treatments, as antibiotics and anti-inflammatory drugs may only provide temporary symptom management without addressing the underlying inflammation and cellular damage.

DMSO has emerged as a potential adjunct therapy for managing Lyme disease and chronic conditions, thanks to its anti-inflammatory, pain-relieving, and detoxifying properties. By penetrating deep into tissues and improving cellular function, DMSO offers a unique approach to reducing symptoms, enhancing immune function, and supporting detoxification in individuals suffering from chronic illness.

Reducing Systemic Inflammation and Joint Pain

One of the hallmark symptoms of chronic Lyme disease and autoimmune conditions is widespread inflammation that affects the joints, muscles, and nervous system. This inflammatory response can lead to debilitating pain, stiffness, and fatigue, often mimicking the symptoms of arthritis or fibromyalgia.

DMSO helps reduce inflammation by:

- Neutralizing inflammatory cytokines, which play a key role in the pain and swelling associated with chronic conditions.
- Enhancing circulation, allowing oxygen and nutrients to reach affected tissues, aiding in cellular repair and detoxification.
- Reducing oxidative stress, preventing further tissue damage and slowing disease progression.

Many individuals with chronic Lyme disease have reported a decrease in joint pain and muscle stiffness after incorporating DMSO into their treatment plans, making it easier to regain mobility and daily function.

Supporting Neurological Function and Cognitive Clarity

Lyme disease and other chronic infections often cause neurological symptoms, including brain fog, memory issues, nerve pain, and cognitive decline. This is due to the inflammatory effects of bacterial infections, immune dysfunction, and oxidative stress in the nervous system.

DMSO offers potential neurological benefits by:

- Crossing the blood-brain barrier, allowing it to deliver anti-inflammatory compounds and antioxidants directly to the brain.
- Reducing nerve inflammation, easing symptoms like neuropathy, tingling, and shooting pains.
- Enhancing mitochondrial function, which plays a critical role in energy production and cognitive function.

Individuals using DMSO therapy for Lyme-related neurological issues have reported improvements in focus, reduced nerve pain, and greater mental clarity, helping them regain cognitive function.

Detoxification and Immune System Support

One of the biggest challenges in chronic Lyme disease and autoimmune conditions is the accumulation of toxins, heavy metals, and microbial byproducts in the body. These substances contribute to chronic inflammation, immune dysfunction, and energy depletion.

DMSO supports detoxification by:

- Binding to heavy metals and toxins, allowing them to be flushed out more efficiently.
- Enhancing lymphatic drainage, helping the body remove cellular waste.
- Improving immune function, allowing the body to better fight chronic infections.

By assisting with detoxification and immune regulation, DMSO may help restore balance in individuals suffering from chronic illnesses, offering them a potential path to better health and symptom relief.

Case Studies on High-Dose Treatment Safety

The use of high-dose DMSO therapy has been a subject of both intrigue and debate in the medical and alternative health communities. While low to moderate doses have been widely recognized for their anti-inflammatory, analgesic, and detoxifying properties, higher doses have been explored for treating chronic diseases, neurological conditions, and advanced inflammation-related disorders.

To understand the safety profile and effectiveness of high-dose DMSO treatment, researchers, practitioners, and patient case studies provide valuable insights. These real-world applications highlight both the potential benefits and risks, offering a clearer picture of how DMSO interacts with the body in more intensive therapeutic settings.

High-Dose DMSO in Chronic Inflammation Management

One of the most well-documented applications of high-dose DMSO therapy has been in patients suffering from chronic inflammatory conditions, such as rheumatoid arthritis, fibromyalgia, and advanced autoimmune disorders.

- **Case Example:** A 52-year-old woman diagnosed with severe rheumatoid arthritis had previously relied on steroids and immunosuppressants to manage her pain and swelling. However, these medications led to digestive issues and long-term dependency concerns. Under medical supervision, she began high-dose DMSO therapy at concentrations of 70% applied topically, twice daily. Within six weeks, she reported a substantial reduction in joint stiffness, improved mobility, and decreased reliance on pharmaceutical drugs.
- **Safety Considerations:** The patient experienced mild skin irritation during the first week but adjusted by using aloe vera as a carrier to dilute the solution slightly. No significant adverse effects were reported beyond the characteristic garlic-like odor associated with DMSO metabolism.

Neurological Recovery and High-Dose DMSO

Neurological conditions such as multiple sclerosis (MS), Parkinson's disease, and traumatic brain injury (TBI) have been explored in alternative medicine circles for DMSO's potential neuroprotective benefits.

- **Case Example:** A 61-year-old male with early-stage Parkinson's disease began a high-dose oral and topical DMSO regimen under the supervision of an integrative physician. The therapy involved oral DMSO diluted in distilled water, along with transdermal applications to the spine and neck area. After three months, his tremors had significantly reduced, and cognitive function improved, as reported by family members and caregivers.
- **Safety Considerations:** The patient reported an initial detox reaction, including mild headaches and increased urination, which subsided after two weeks. Hydration and mineral supplementation were emphasized to support the detoxification process.

Cancer Support and High-Dose DMSO Protocols

While not a standalone cancer treatment, some patients have used high-dose DMSO as an adjunct therapy, often in combination with high-dose vitamin C and oxygen therapy to enhance cellular oxygenation and detoxification.

- **Case Example:** A 47-year-old woman with stage III breast cancer integrated DMSO with her chemotherapy regimen, as recommended by an integrative oncology specialist. She received intravenous vitamin C with DMSO to enhance absorption and reduce chemotherapy side effects. Over time, she experienced less nausea, better energy levels, and reduced neuropathy symptoms compared to her previous chemotherapy cycles.
- **Safety Considerations:** Careful medical monitoring was essential, as DMSO can enhance the absorption of other substances, including chemotherapy drugs, requiring precise dosage adjustments to avoid toxicity.

These case studies demonstrate that while high-dose DMSO therapy shows promising results, it requires careful administration, supervision, and patient-specific adjustments to ensure safety and effectiveness.

CHAPTER 26
COMBINING DMSO WITH OTHER ADVANCED THERAPIES

Synergistic Effects with Ozone, Hydrogen Peroxide, and Chelation Therapy

DMSO is well known for its anti-inflammatory, analgesic, and detoxifying properties, but its potential is amplified when combined with other biological therapies that support cellular health and detoxification. Among the most promising synergies are its interactions with ozone therapy, hydrogen peroxide therapy, and chelation therapy—three modalities known for their oxidative and detoxifying effects. These therapies work in tandem with DMSO to enhance oxygen delivery, eliminate toxins, and support systemic healing.

Ozone Therapy and DMSO: A Potent Combination for Oxygenation

Ozone therapy involves the controlled administration of ozone (O_3), a highly reactive form of oxygen, to improve circulation, immunity, and cellular respiration. It has been widely used in integrative medicine for conditions like chronic infections, cardiovascular disease, and autoimmune disorders.

DMSO enhances the effects of ozone therapy in several key ways:

- **Oxygen delivery:** DMSO increases the penetration of ozone into tissues, ensuring that oxygen reaches deeper cellular levels.
- **Antimicrobial synergy:** Both ozone and DMSO have potent antimicrobial properties, making them effective in addressing bacterial, viral, and fungal infections.
- **Detoxification support:** Ozone therapy triggers the release of toxins at the cellular level, and DMSO helps transport these toxins out of the body more efficiently.

Patients who have undergone DMSO-ozone therapy report improved energy levels, enhanced detoxification, and faster recovery from chronic infections, particularly Lyme disease, mold toxicity, and viral illnesses.

Hydrogen Peroxide Therapy and DMSO: Enhancing Cellular Cleansing

Hydrogen peroxide (H_2O_2) therapy is based on the principle that controlled oxidative stress can stimulate cellular detoxification, enhance immune function, and improve oxygenation. When administered in appropriate doses, hydrogen peroxide helps break down pathogens, neutralize toxins, and increase metabolic efficiency.

The synergy between DMSO and hydrogen peroxide lies in their ability to amplify oxidative therapy without excessive cellular damage:

- **Deep tissue penetration:** DMSO helps carry hydrogen peroxide deeper into tissues, improving its ability to target hypoxic (low-oxygen) areas of the body.
- **Immune modulation:** Hydrogen peroxide stimulates the production of white blood cells, while DMSO helps reduce the inflammatory damage caused by chronic infections.
- **Support for oxidative stress balance:** While hydrogen peroxide induces mild oxidative stress, DMSO provides antioxidant benefits that prevent excessive tissue damage.

Patients using DMSO with hydrogen peroxide therapy have reported benefits in chronic fatigue syndrome, immune dysfunction, and detoxification-related symptoms.

Chelation Therapy and DMSO: A Dual Detoxification Approach

Chelation therapy is used to remove heavy metals and toxic elements from the bloodstream, typically through intravenous EDTA (ethylenediaminetetraacetic acid) or natural chelators like alpha-lipoic acid and zeolite.

DMSO enhances the effectiveness of chelation therapy in several ways:

- **Binding and transporting metals:** DMSO has the unique ability to bind to heavy metals and facilitate their excretion through urine, sweat, and feces.
- **Reducing oxidative damage:** Heavy metal toxicity generates free radicals that contribute to inflammation and cellular dysfunction—DMSO's antioxidant properties help counteract this damage.
- **Improving circulation:** Chelation therapy often mobilizes toxins from deep tissue reservoirs, and DMSO enhances circulatory function, ensuring effective elimination.

Many individuals undergoing chelation therapy with DMSO support experience faster recovery from metal toxicity, improved cognitive function, and relief from chronic inflammatory symptoms.

By combining DMSO with these advanced therapies, individuals can accelerate detoxification, support oxygenation, and enhance immune resilience, making it a valuable integrative tool for long-term healing and disease prevention.

Emerging Research on Future Applications

As DMSO continues to be studied in both clinical and experimental settings, researchers are uncovering new applications that could revolutionize pain management, neurodegenerative disease treatment, regenerative medicine, and oncology support. While DMSO has been widely recognized for its anti-inflammatory, analgesic, and detoxifying properties, cutting-edge research is pushing its potential even further. Scientists are now exploring its role in drug delivery, stem cell therapy, tissue regeneration, and even genetic medicine.

DMSO as a Next-Generation Drug Carrier

One of the most exciting areas of research focuses on DMSO's ability to act as a biological carrier, enhancing drug absorption and targeted delivery.

- **Improving chemotherapy efficacy:** Scientists are investigating how DMSO can enhance the penetration of chemotherapy drugs into cancerous tissues while simultaneously reducing systemic toxicity. This approach may help lower drug dosages while maintaining therapeutic effects.
- **Transdermal drug administration:** Since DMSO penetrates the skin within seconds, it is being explored as a carrier for transdermal pain relief and hormonal therapies. This research aims to provide needle-free medication delivery, particularly beneficial for patients with chronic pain, hormonal imbalances, or gastrointestinal sensitivities.
- **Targeting brain diseases:** Researchers are studying whether DMSO can cross the blood-brain barrier more efficiently than existing drug carriers, offering a potential way to deliver neuroprotective compounds directly into the central nervous system. This could have significant implications for Alzheimer's, Parkinson's, and other neurodegenerative conditions.

DMSO and Stem Cell Therapy

Another promising area of exploration is the use of DMSO in stem cell preservation and delivery. Stem cells are highly sensitive to environmental conditions, and researchers have found that DMSO helps preserve their viability during storage and transplantation.

- **Enhancing stem cell survival:** Cryopreservation with DMSO protects stem cells from oxidative stress, allowing them to be more effectively used in regenerative medicine.
- **Optimizing stem cell therapy for tissue repair:** Clinical trials are investigating whether DMSO can improve the integration of stem cells into damaged tissues, enhancing healing in orthopedic injuries, cardiac repair, and nerve regeneration.
- **Reducing transplant rejection:** Some studies suggest that DMSO's anti-inflammatory properties may reduce immune system overactivity, lowering the risk of stem cell transplant rejection in patients with autoimmune diseases.

DMSO in Genetic and Epigenetic Medicine

Researchers are also examining DMSO's effects on DNA repair, gene expression, and epigenetic regulation, which could open new frontiers in genetic medicine.

- **DNA stability and protection:** Studies indicate that DMSO may help protect DNA from oxidative damage, reducing the risk of mutations that contribute to cancer and degenerative diseases.
- **Gene therapy applications:** Preliminary research suggests that DMSO may enhance gene editing efficiency, making it a potential adjunct therapy in CRISPR-based genetic treatments.
- **Epigenetic regulation:** Some studies propose that DMSO influences methylation and gene expression, which may play a role in turning off inflammatory genes or activating cellular repair pathways.

With these emerging discoveries, DMSO is on the path to becoming a central player in future medical advancements, expanding beyond its traditional uses and into cutting-edge therapies that may transform modern healthcare.

BOOK 14
THE CONTROVERSY SURROUNDING DMSO

CHAPTER 27
WHY DMSO REMAINS CONTROVERSIAL

The Role of the FDA and Pharmaceutical Industry

DMSO has been at the center of a long-standing controversy, not because of its effectiveness, but because of the complex interplay between regulatory agencies and the pharmaceutical industry. Despite decades of research and countless anecdotal reports confirming DMSO's therapeutic benefits, it remains largely unapproved for widespread medical use in the United States. This raises an important question: why is a safe, inexpensive, and highly effective compound not readily available to the public? The answer lies in the intricate dynamics between the FDA, pharmaceutical companies, and the regulatory process that governs drug approval.

The FDA's Stance on DMSO

The Food and Drug Administration (FDA) plays a crucial role in evaluating and approving medical treatments for public use. While this regulatory oversight is necessary to ensure drug safety and efficacy, many argue that DMSO has been unjustly scrutinized compared to other pharmaceuticals with far greater risks.

- **Limited approvals:** The FDA has only approved DMSO for interstitial cystitis (a painful bladder condition), despite evidence suggesting its benefits extend to arthritis, neurological disorders, inflammation, and even cancer therapy.
- **Stringent testing requirements:** Unlike patented drugs that receive billions in funding for clinical trials, DMSO, as a naturally occurring compound, lacks corporate financial backing to push it through the costly FDA approval process.
- **Inconsistent regulation:** While the FDA restricts DMSO for most medical applications, it is widely used in veterinary medicine, laboratory research, and industrial applications, demonstrating a double standard in its classification.

This selective approval has led to frustration within the medical community, especially among practitioners who have witnessed DMSO's effectiveness in pain relief, wound healing, and chronic disease management.

The Pharmaceutical Industry's Role in Suppressing DMSO

Pharmaceutical companies operate for profit, and the existence of a low-cost, natural, and highly effective compound like DMSO poses a direct threat to their business model. Unlike synthetic drugs that can be patented, DMSO has been in the public domain for decades, meaning that no single company can monopolize its production and distribution.

- **Lack of financial incentive:** Since DMSO cannot be patented, pharmaceutical companies have little motivation to fund large-scale clinical trials, making FDA approval financially impractical.
- **Threat to lucrative drug markets:** If widely adopted, DMSO could replace billions of dollars' worth of prescription medications, including NSAIDs, opioids, corticosteroids, and chemotherapy support drugs.
- **Historical suppression:** In the 1960s, promising research on DMSO's medical applications was abruptly halted following pressure from pharmaceutical interests, leading to decades of regulatory red tape.

The suppression of low-cost natural treatments in favor of profitable patented drugs is a recurring theme in medical history, and DMSO is just one example of a therapy that has been pushed to the fringes despite its potential to transform healthcare.

How This Affects Patients Today

As a result of this regulatory and corporate resistance, patients who could benefit immensely from DMSO are left with limited options:

- Turning to alternative medicine practitioners who operate outside the FDA-regulated system.
- Importing pharmaceutical-grade DMSO from countries where it is legally available for more than just interstitial cystitis.
- Using industrial-grade DMSO, which is not intended for human consumption but remains one of the few accessible sources.

This ongoing controversy highlights the need for more independent research, medical advocacy, and patient awareness to push for a reassessment of DMSO's place in modern medicine.

Addressing Common Myths and Misconceptions

DMSO has been the subject of controversy and misinformation for decades. Despite its well-documented anti-inflammatory, analgesic, and healing properties, misconceptions have prevented it from becoming a mainstream treatment. Much of the skepticism surrounding DMSO stems from outdated research, regulatory restrictions, and a lack of public awareness. Here, we'll address some of the most persistent myths and clarify the scientific realities behind this misunderstood compound.

Myth 1: DMSO Is Only a Harsh Industrial Solvent

One of the most common misconceptions is that DMSO is unsafe for human use because it is widely used as an industrial solvent. While it's true that DMSO has applications in paint stripping, antifreeze, and chemical processing, this fact alone does not make it inherently dangerous.

- **Reality:** Many pharmaceutical compounds, including aspirin and acetaminophen, have industrial applications yet remain safe and effective for human consumption when properly formulated.
- Medical-grade DMSO is highly purified, eliminating the contaminants present in industrial versions. It has been used in medical settings for decades, including in FDA-approved treatments for interstitial cystitis and cryopreservation of stem cells.

Myth 2: DMSO Is a Dangerous, Untested Chemical

Skeptics often claim that DMSO lacks sufficient scientific research and is therefore too risky to use. This perception is largely based on a lack of awareness rather than factual evidence.

- **Reality:** Over 1,000 scientific studies have investigated the safety and efficacy of DMSO, including research from prestigious institutions like Stanford University, the Cleveland Clinic, and the National Institutes of Health (NIH).
- Clinical trials in multiple countries have demonstrated DMSO's powerful effects in reducing inflammation, accelerating wound healing, and protecting nerve cells.
- While early studies in the 1960s raised concerns about eye toxicity in high doses, modern research has disproven these fears, confirming that DMSO is safe when used correctly.

Myth 3: DMSO Causes a Garlic Smell Because It's Toxic

One of the most misunderstood aspects of DMSO is its ability to cause a garlic-like odor on the breath and skin. Some assume that this reaction is a sign of toxicity, leading them to question its safety.

- **Reality:** The garlic-like smell occurs because DMSO rapidly penetrates tissues and metabolizes into dimethyl sulfide (DMS), a natural sulfur compound.
- This is not a sign of toxicity—it is simply a metabolic byproduct and varies from person to person. Some individuals barely notice the odor, while others experience it more intensely.
- Sulfur-based compounds like onions, garlic, and cruciferous vegetables can produce similar effects, but they are not considered harmful.

Myth 4: DMSO Is Unsafe Because It Can Carry Harmful Substances Into the Body

A valid concern about DMSO is its ability to transport molecules through the skin and into the bloodstream. Some fear that this could introduce harmful chemicals into the body.

- **Reality:** While DMSO does enhance absorption, this property is only a risk if combined with toxic substances.
- Medical professionals and researchers safely use DMSO by ensuring that the skin and surrounding environment are clean before application.
- Many FDA-approved transdermal medications use DMSO's unique absorption properties to enhance drug delivery.

Myth 5: If DMSO Were Truly Effective, It Would Be Approved for More Conditions

Many assume that if DMSO were a legitimate treatment, the FDA and pharmaceutical companies would have pushed for its widespread approval. The fact that it is not commonly prescribed leads some to dismiss it as ineffective or unsafe.

- **Reality:** The regulatory and financial barriers surrounding natural and non-patentable compounds prevent many effective therapies from becoming mainstream.
- Since DMSO is a naturally occurring substance, no pharmaceutical company can patent it and profit exclusively, making large-scale clinical trials financially unappealing.
- The FDA has approved DMSO for specific medical uses, and other countries—including Russia, Canada, and parts of Europe—allow broader medical applications.

By debunking these myths and understanding the scientific reality, individuals can make informed decisions about whether DMSO is right for them. Despite its controversial reputation, its potential in natural healing and alternative medicine remains undeniable.

CHAPTER 28

THE LEGAL AND ETHICAL LANDSCAPE OF DMSO

Regulations in the U.S. and Worldwide

The legal landscape of DMSO is complex, varying significantly between countries. While some nations recognize its therapeutic potential and allow medical applications, others restrict its use due to historical concerns, lack of financial incentives for large-scale studies, or regulatory inertia. Understanding these regulations and policies is crucial for those seeking to use DMSO for personal health, veterinary care, or alternative treatments.

The U.S. Regulatory Status: A Conflicted Position

In the United States, DMSO exists in a regulatory gray area. The Food and Drug Administration (FDA) has approved its use for a limited number of medical conditions, yet it remains unapproved for many other therapeutic applications, despite extensive research supporting its benefits.

- **FDA-Approved Uses:**
- **Interstitial cystitis treatment:** DMSO is officially sanctioned for bladder inflammation relief under the brand name Rimso-50.
- **Cryopreservation of stem cells and organ tissues:** It is used in medical research and transplantation medicine.
- **Unapproved but widely used applications:**
- Many alternative health practitioners and individuals use DMSO for pain relief, inflammation control, and tissue healing, even though these applications lack formal FDA approval.
- **Legality for purchase and personal use:**
- DMSO is legally available in the U.S. as an industrial solvent but is not labeled for medical use.
- Doctors cannot prescribe it for conditions outside of its approved indications, leading many users to seek over-the-counter (OTC) alternatives.

The FDA's reluctance to expand approval for DMSO's medical applications has fueled skepticism among its proponents. Many argue that the lack of financial incentives—since DMSO is naturally occurring and cannot be patented—has discouraged pharmaceutical companies from funding large-scale clinical trials.

DMSO Regulations in Canada and Europe

Outside the U.S., regulatory attitudes toward DMSO vary widely:

- **Canada:**
- DMSO is not approved as a drug but is available as an industrial solvent.
- Some naturopathic practitioners recommend it off-label, and veterinary use is more widely accepted.
- **European Union (EU):**
- Some European countries, including Germany and France, allow limited medicinal use of DMSO under specific conditions.
- It is often incorporated into compounded medications for pain management and inflammation reduction.
- **United Kingdom:**
- DMSO is not classified as a pharmaceutical drug, meaning it is available for purchase but lacks official medical approval.
- **Russia and Eastern Europe:**
- Russia has been one of the strongest proponents of DMSO in medical treatments.
- It is used for anti-inflammatory purposes, wound healing, and even neurological recovery therapies.

DMSO Regulations in Latin America and Asia

Regulations in Latin America and Asia tend to be more lenient compared to the U.S. and Western Europe.

- **Mexico:**
- DMSO is widely used in alternative and holistic medicine, particularly in cancer clinics that offer integrative treatments.
- It is often combined with other natural therapies and used in injectable forms.
- **Brazil and Argentina:**
- Similar to the U.S., DMSO is available but primarily labeled as an industrial product rather than a pharmaceutical treatment.
- **China and Japan:**
- In China, herbal medicine practitioners have experimented with DMSO, but regulatory approval remains limited.
- Japan has conducted some research on DMSO, but medical use is not widespread.

Why the Regulations Differ Globally

The discrepancy in global regulations surrounding DMSO can be attributed to:

1. **Lack of patentability** – Since DMSO is a **naturally occurring compound**, pharmaceutical

companies **cannot secure exclusive rights**, making large-scale clinical trials **financially unappealing**.

2. **Historic safety concerns** – Early studies in the 1960s raised **toxicity fears**, particularly regarding **eye damage**, although later research largely debunked these concerns.
3. **Influence of pharmaceutical interests** – Countries with **strong pharmaceutical lobbying efforts** tend to have **stricter regulations**, as DMSO poses a **low-cost alternative** to many expensive medications.

Despite these challenges, DMSO continues to gain traction as new research and public demand push for greater accessibility in medical applications worldwide.

Ensuring Safe and Responsible Use

While DMSO offers a wide range of therapeutic benefits, ensuring its safe and responsible use is crucial. Because it has the unique ability to penetrate the skin and carry substances directly into the bloodstream, improper handling can lead to unintended contamination or side effects. Understanding the best practices, appropriate dosages, and necessary precautions is essential for anyone using DMSO for personal health, veterinary applications, or alternative treatments.

Choosing High-Quality, Medical-Grade DMSO

Not all DMSO products are created equal. Since DMSO is widely available as an industrial solvent, some products may contain chemical impurities or be stored in non-medical-grade containers, which could pose serious health risks.

- **Look for purity certifications:** The highest-quality DMSO is 99.99% pure, labeled as medical- or pharmaceutical-grade.
- **Avoid industrial-grade formulations:** These may contain toxic byproducts that are unsafe for human or animal use.
- **Check the storage container:** Glass is the best option, as DMSO can leach chemicals from plastic containers, potentially introducing harmful substances into the body.

Proper Application Techniques

Because DMSO acts as a carrier, it can introduce contaminants into the bloodstream if applied incorrectly. To minimize risks:

- Always wash your hands thoroughly before and after handling DMSO.
- Use clean, sterile materials (such as cotton swabs or glass droppers) to apply the solution.
- Avoid synthetic fabrics and lotions in the application area, as DMSO can absorb chemicals from these materials.
- Wait for the area to dry completely before covering it with clothing.

Determining the Right Concentration

DMSO is often diluted to different concentrations depending on the intended use. Using too strong of a solution may cause skin irritation or discomfort, while overly diluted solutions may be less effective.

- **Typical concentrations for topical use:**
- **50-70% DMSO:** Common for joint pain, inflammation, and muscle injuries.
- **25-50% DMSO:** Suitable for sensitive areas or prolonged use.
- **10-20% DMSO:** Recommended for facial applications or delicate skin.
- **Avoid high concentrations on delicate skin:** Using 100% DMSO directly on the skin can cause burning, redness, and irritation.

Recognizing Potential Side Effects

Although DMSO is well tolerated by most users, some side effects may occur, especially when used improperly or in excessive amounts.

- **Common side effects:**
- A garlic-like odor on the breath or skin (a temporary but well-documented effect).
- Mild skin irritation, redness, or itching.
- Temporary headaches or dizziness in some individuals.
- **Rare but serious concerns:**
- **Eye irritation:** High doses have been linked to temporary vision changes in some studies.
- **Contaminant absorption:** If applied incorrectly, DMSO can carry harmful substances into the bloodstream.

If any severe allergic reactions or persistent side effects occur, discontinuing use and consulting a healthcare professional is advised.

Safe Use for Different Populations

While DMSO is generally safe for adult use, there are certain groups who should take extra precautions or avoid its use altogether.

- **Pregnant or breastfeeding women:** DMSO has not been extensively studied in pregnancy, and its ability to cross biological barriers raises safety concerns.
- **Children:** Due to their sensitive skin and developing bodies, pediatric use of DMSO should only be considered under professional guidance.
- **Individuals with liver or kidney conditions:** Because DMSO is metabolized in the liver and excreted through the kidneys, those with pre-existing conditions should consult a medical expert before using it.

Interactions with Medications and Supplements

One of the most overlooked aspects of DMSO is its interaction with other substances. Because it enhances absorption, it can increase the potency of medications, herbs, and supplements, potentially leading to unintended effects.

- **Anti-inflammatory drugs (NSAIDs, steroids):** DMSO may amplify their effects, increasing the risk of gastric irritation or toxicity.
- **Blood thinners (warfarin, aspirin):** DMSO may enhance blood-thinning properties, potentially raising the risk of bruising or bleeding.
- **Alcohol and caffeine:** Using DMSO with stimulants or depressants may intensify their effects, leading to stronger reactions.

Anyone using prescription medications should consult a healthcare provider before incorporating DMSO into their routine.

Legal and Ethical Considerations for Responsible Use

Since DMSO is not approved for all therapeutic uses, it is important to exercise caution when using or recommending it.

- **Be transparent with medical professionals:** While some doctors may be unfamiliar with DMSO, openly discussing its use can help prevent unwanted interactions.
- **Avoid exaggerated claims:** While many users swear by its healing benefits, DMSO is not a cure-all. Misrepresenting its effects could lead to misinformation or unrealistic expectations.
- **Stay informed on evolving research:** Because DMSO remains a controversial compound, staying updated on new studies, regulatory changes, and expert opinions can help ensure safe and responsible use.

By following these best practices, individuals can maximize the benefits of DMSO while minimizing potential risks, ensuring its safe and effective integration into health and wellness routines.

BOOK 15
DMSO REMEDIES FOR EYE HEALTH (CATARACTS, VISION RESTORATION)

CHAPTER 29
TARGETED DMSO APPLICATIONS FOR VISION SUPPORT

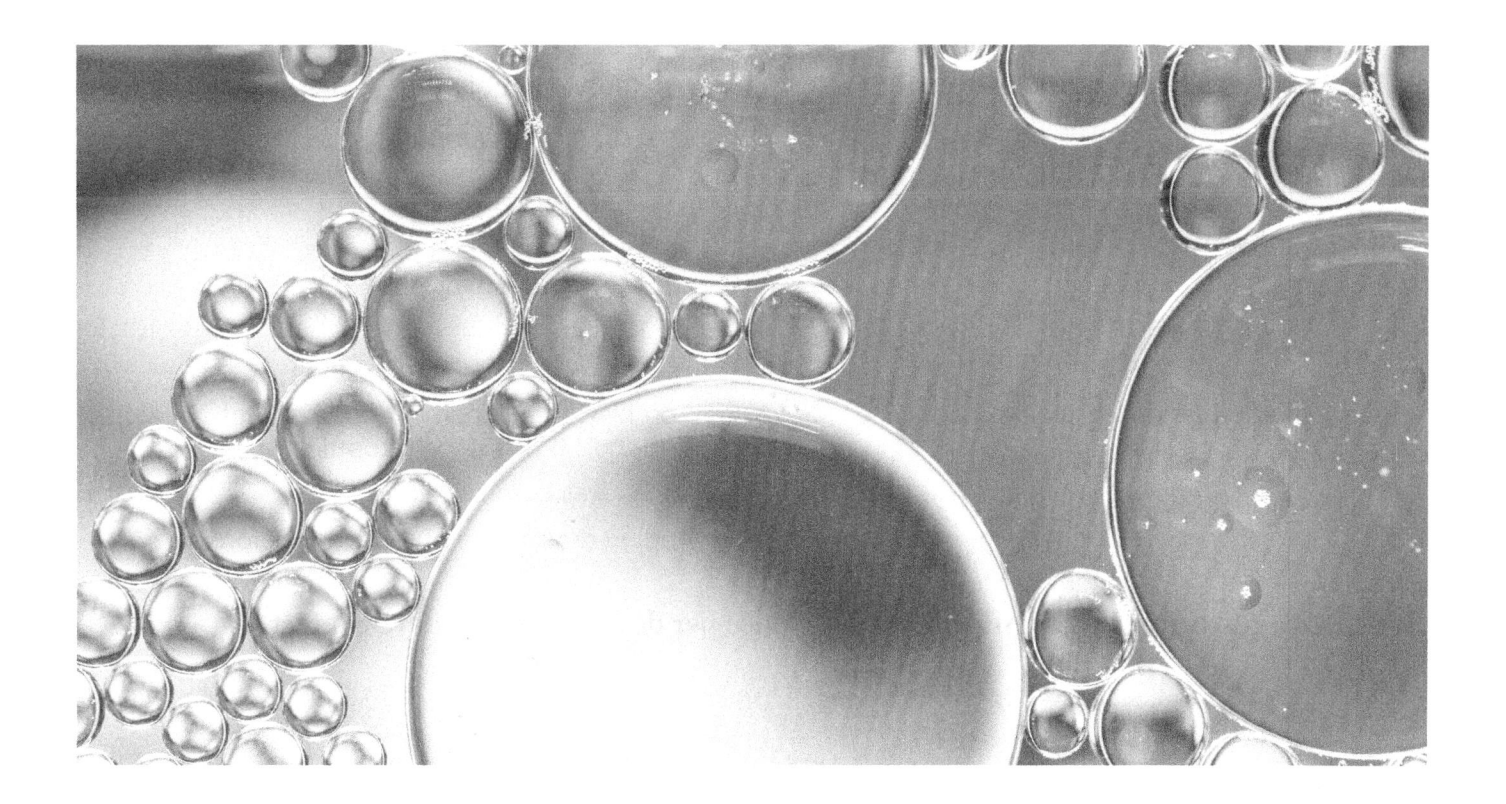

DMSO Eye Compress for Cataract Clarity

INGREDIENTS

- DMSO (99% pure, diluted to 30%)
- Sterile distilled water
- Organic cotton pads

PREPARATION

1. Mix 3 parts sterile distilled water with 1 part DMSO in a clean glass container.
2. Soak a cotton pad in the solution and gently place it over the closed eyelid.
3. Leave for 5-10 minutes, then remove and rinse the eye area with sterile water.

Safe Dosages and Usage Guidelines: Use once per day, preferably before bedtime. Avoid direct contact with the eye.

Aloe Vera & DMSO Blend for Dry Eyes Relief

INGREDIENTS

- Organic aloe vera gel
- DMSO (99% pure, diluted to 40%)
- Sterile saline solution

PREPARATION

1. Mix 1 teaspoon of aloe vera gel with 3 drops of diluted DMSO.
2. Add 1 teaspoon of sterile saline and stir gently.
3. Apply a drop to the outer eyelid and massage lightly.

Safe Dosages and Usage Guidelines: Use up to twice daily. Do not apply directly inside the eye.

Castor Oil & DMSO Solution for Retinal Support

INGREDIENTS

- Cold-pressed organic castor oil
- DMSO (99% pure, diluted to 30%)
- Sterile dropper bottle

PREPARATION

1. Combine 1 teaspoon of castor oil with 5 drops of diluted DMSO in a sterile bottle.
2. Shake well before each use.
3. Apply 1 drop to the outer eyelid before sleep.

Safe Dosages and Usage Guidelines: Use once per day. Avoid direct eye contact.

Herbal DMSO Rinse for Eye Fatigue and Strain

INGREDIENTS

- Chamomile tea (cooled)
- DMSO (99% pure, diluted to 30%)
- Sterile saline solution

PREPARATION

1. Brew chamomile tea and allow it to cool completely.
2. Mix 1 tablespoon of tea with 5 drops of diluted DMSO.
3. Use as an eye rinse with a sterile dropper.

Safe Dosages and Usage Guidelines: Use once daily. Ensure the solution is fresh before each use.

Vitamin C & DMSO Eye Pad for Oxidative Stress Reduction

INGREDIENTS

- Buffered vitamin C powder
- DMSO (99% pure, diluted to 30%)
- Sterile water

PREPARATION

1. Dissolve 1/8 teaspoon of vitamin C powder in 1 teaspoon of sterile water.
2. Add 5 drops of diluted DMSO and soak a cotton pad.
3. Apply over closed eyelids for 10 minutes.

Safe Dosages and Usage Guidelines: Use up to 3 times per week. Do not apply inside the eye.

MSM & DMSO Eye Drop Alternative for Lubrication

INGREDIENTS

- MSM powder
- DMSO (99% pure, diluted to 20%)
- Sterile saline solution

PREPARATION

1. Dissolve 1/4 teaspoon of MSM powder in 1 tablespoon of sterile saline.
2. Add 3 drops of diluted DMSO and shake well.
3. Apply 1 drop to the outer eyelid.

Safe Dosages and Usage Guidelines: Use once daily. Avoid direct eye contact.

Bilberry Extract & DMSO Topical Application for Vision Enhancement

INGREDIENTS

- Bilberry extract (liquid)
- DMSO (99% pure, diluted to 40%)
- Sterile cotton swabs

PREPARATION

1. Mix 1 teaspoon of bilberry extract with 5 drops of diluted DMSO.
2. Dip a cotton swab into the mixture and apply around the eyes.
3. Let absorb for 5 minutes, then rinse if needed.

Safe Dosages and Usage Guidelines: Use up to twice per day. Avoid direct eye contact.

Chamomile & DMSO Cold Compress for Reducing Eye Inflammation

INGREDIENTS
- Chamomile tea (cooled)
- DMSO (99% pure, diluted to 30%)
- Sterile gauze

PREPARATION
1. Soak sterile gauze in cooled chamomile tea.
2. Add 5 drops of diluted DMSO.
3. Apply as a cold compress for 10 minutes.

Safe Dosages and Usage Guidelines: Use as needed for inflammation relief.

DMSO & Saline Wash for Gentle Eye Detoxification

INGREDIENTS
- DMSO (99% pure, diluted to 20%)
- Sterile saline solution
- Sterile dropper bottle

PREPARATION
1. Mix 1 part DMSO with 4 parts sterile saline in a dropper bottle.
2. Shake well before each use.
3. Use as a gentle rinse by applying drops to the outer eye area.

Safe Dosages and Usage Guidelines: Use once daily for mild detoxification.

Coconut Water & DMSO Eye Soothing Formula

INGREDIENTS
- Fresh coconut water (sterile)
- DMSO (99% pure, diluted to 20%)
- Sterile cotton pads

PREPARATION
1. Mix 1 tablespoon of coconut water with 5 drops of diluted DMSO.
2. Soak a cotton pad and place over closed eyelids.
3. Leave on for 5 minutes, then discard.

Safe Dosages and Usage Guidelines: Use up to twice daily for eye hydration.

BOOK 16

DMSO REMEDIES FOR DIGESTIVE DISORDERS (IBS, CROHN'S DISEASE)

CHAPTER 30

DMSO PROTOCOLS FOR GUT HEALTH AND DIGESTIVE RECOVERY

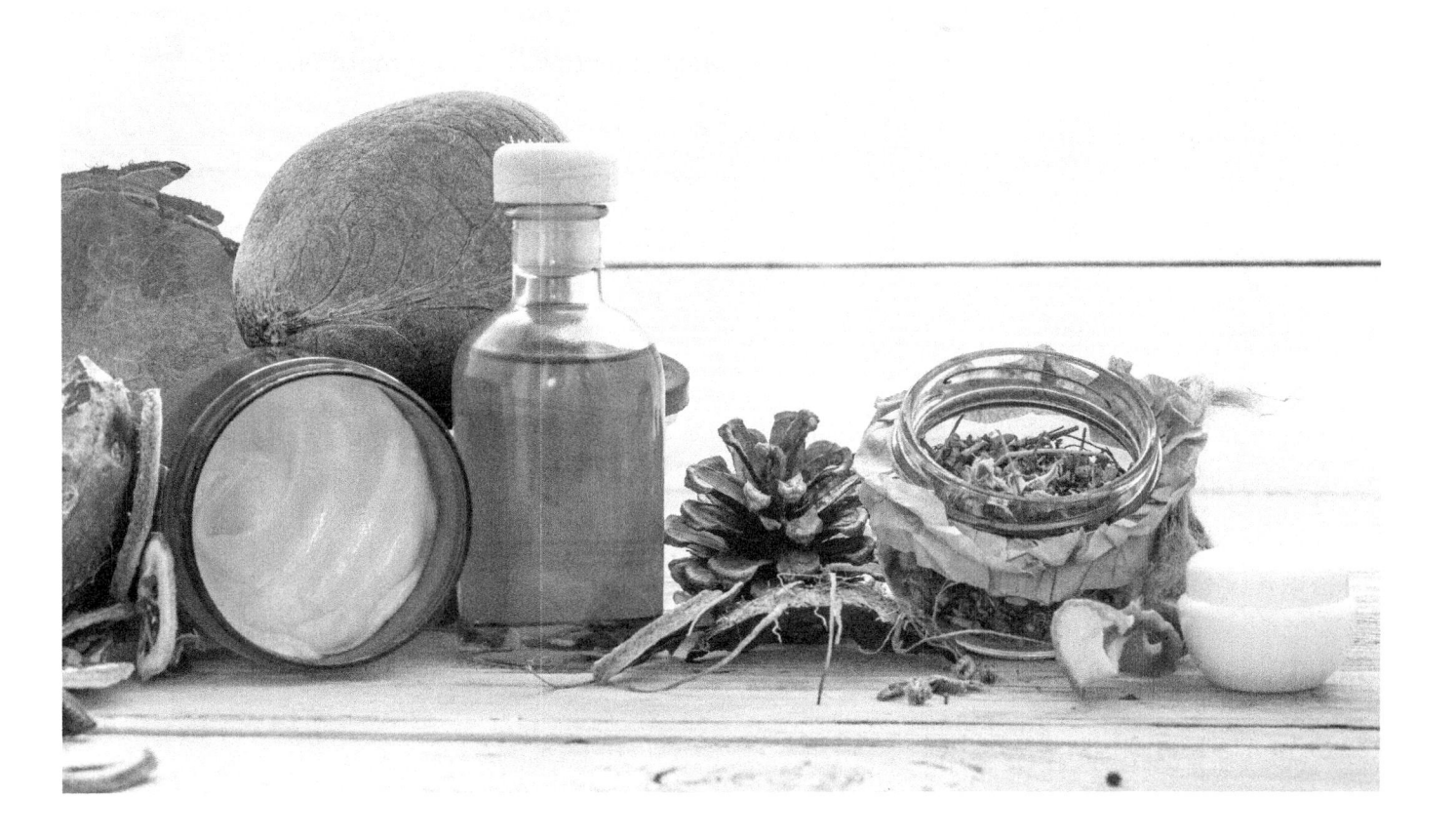

DMSO & Aloe Vera Drink for Gut Lining Support

INGREDIENTS

- Organic aloe vera juice
- DMSO (99% pure, diluted to 30%)
- Filtered water

PREPARATION

1. Mix 1 tablespoon of aloe vera juice with 5 drops of diluted DMSO.
2. Add 1/2 cup of filtered water and stir well.
3. Drink slowly on an empty stomach.

Safe Dosages and Usage Guidelines: Consume once daily before meals for digestive support.

Chamomile & DMSO Infusion for IBS Symptom Relief

INGREDIENTS

- Dried chamomile flowers
- DMSO (99% pure, diluted to 30%)
- Hot filtered water

PREPARATION

1. Steep 1 teaspoon of dried chamomile flowers in 1 cup of hot water for 10 minutes.
2. Strain and let it cool to lukewarm temperature.
3. Add 5 drops of diluted DMSO and stir well.

Safe Dosages and Usage Guidelines: Drink once daily to ease IBS symptoms.

Slippery Elm & DMSO Blend for Soothing Intestinal Inflammation

INGREDIENTS

- Slippery elm powder
- DMSO (99% pure, diluted to 30%)
- Filtered water

PREPARATION

1. Mix 1 teaspoon of slippery elm powder with 1/2 cup of warm water.
2. Add 5 drops of diluted DMSO and stir until fully blended.
3. Let it sit for 2 minutes before drinking.

Safe Dosages and Usage Guidelines: Take once per day to soothe intestinal inflammation.

Coconut Water & DMSO Hydration Therapy for Digestive Balance

INGREDIENTS

- Organic coconut water
- DMSO (99% pure, diluted to 30%)

PREPARATION

1. Pour 1/2 cup of coconut water into a glass.
2. Add 5 drops of diluted DMSO and stir well.

Safe Dosages and Usage Guidelines: Drink once daily to support hydration and digestion.

DMSO & Marshmallow Root Formula for Ulcer Protection

INGREDIENTS
- Marshmallow root tea
- DMSO (99% pure, diluted to 30%)

PREPARATION
1. Brew 1 cup of marshmallow root tea and let it cool to lukewarm.
2. Add 5 drops of diluted DMSO and stir well.

Safe Dosages and Usage Guidelines: Drink once daily to protect the stomach lining.

Peppermint Oil & DMSO Stomach Massage for Bloating Reduction

INGREDIENTS
- DMSO (99% pure, diluted to 50%)
- Peppermint essential oil
- Carrier oil (such as coconut or olive oil)

PREPARATION
1. Mix 1 teaspoon of carrier oil with 5 drops of DMSO.
2. Add 2 drops of peppermint essential oil and blend well.
3. Gently massage onto the stomach in circular motions.

Safe Dosages and Usage Guidelines: Apply once daily to reduce bloating and discomfort.

Probiotic Yogurt & DMSO Topical Application for Gut Microbiome Support

INGREDIENTS
- Plain probiotic yogurt
- DMSO (99% pure, diluted to 30%)

PREPARATION
1. Mix 1 tablespoon of probiotic yogurt with 5 drops of diluted DMSO.
2. Apply gently to the lower abdomen and leave on for 10 minutes before rinsing.

Safe Dosages and Usage Guidelines: Use once per day to promote gut microbiome balance.

Ginger & DMSO Compress for Reducing Abdominal Discomfort

INGREDIENTS

- Fresh ginger juice
- DMSO (99% pure, diluted to 30%)
- Warm water
- Clean cloth

PREPARATION

1. Soak the clean cloth in warm water and wring out excess liquid.
2. Mix 1 teaspoon of ginger juice with 5 drops of diluted DMSO.
3. Apply the mixture to the cloth and place it on the abdomen for 15 minutes.

Safe Dosages and Usage Guidelines: Use once daily to alleviate digestive discomfort.

Bone Broth & DMSO Elixir for Intestinal Healing

INGREDIENTS

- Warm homemade bone broth
- DMSO (99% pure, diluted to 30%)

PREPARATION

1. Pour 1/2 cup of warm bone broth into a glass.
2. Add 5 drops of diluted DMSO and stir well.

Safe Dosages and Usage Guidelines: Drink once daily for gut healing.

Licorice Root & DMSO Solution for Acid Reflux Control

INGREDIENTS

- Licorice root tea
- DMSO (99% pure, diluted to 30%)

PREPARATION

1. Brew 1 cup of licorice root tea and let it cool slightly.
2. Add 5 drops of diluted DMSO and stir well.

Safe Dosages and Usage Guidelines: Consume once daily to soothe acid reflux.

BOOK 17
DMSO REMEDIES FOR RESPIRATORY HEALTH (ASTHMA, COPD)

CHAPTER 31

STRENGTHENING LUNG FUNCTION WITH DMSO THERAPIES

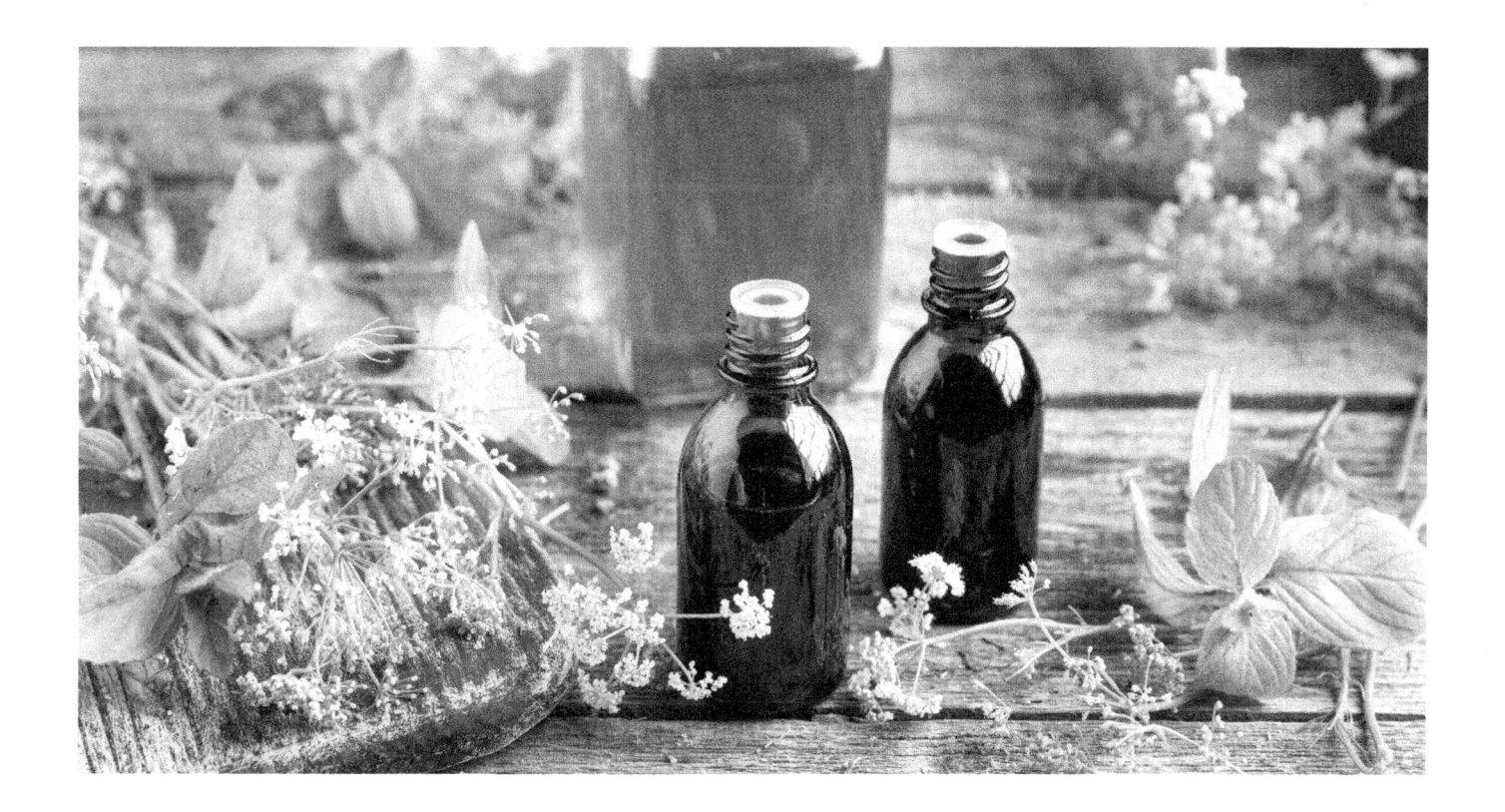

DMSO & Eucalyptus Steam Inhalation for Clearer Airways

INGREDIENTS

- DMSO (99% pure, diluted to 30%)
- Eucalyptus essential oil
- Hot water

PREPARATION

1. Pour 2 cups of hot water into a bowl.
2. Add 3 drops of eucalyptus essential oil.
3. Add 5 drops of diluted DMSO and stir gently.
4. Inhale the steam by placing a towel over your head for 10 minutes.

Safe Dosages and Usage Guidelines: Use once daily to support clear airways.

Honey & DMSO Chest Rub for Respiratory Comfort

INGREDIENTS

- Raw organic honey
- DMSO (99% pure, diluted to 50%)

PREPARATION

1. Mix 1 tablespoon of honey with 5 drops of diluted DMSO.
2. Gently rub the mixture onto the chest area.

Safe Dosages and Usage Guidelines: Apply once daily to promote respiratory comfort.

Peppermint & DMSO Vapor Rub for Sinus and Lung Relief

INGREDIENTS

- Peppermint essential oil
- DMSO (99% pure, diluted to 50%)
- Carrier oil (e.g., coconut or olive oil)

PREPARATION

1. Combine 1 teaspoon of carrier oil with 5 drops of diluted DMSO.
2. Add 2 drops of peppermint essential oil and mix well.
3. Massage onto the chest and neck area.

Safe Dosages and Usage Guidelines: Use once daily to relieve sinus and lung discomfort.

Saline & DMSO Nebulizer Solution for Lung Hydration

INGREDIENTS

- Sterile saline solution
- DMSO (99% pure, diluted to 30%)

PREPARATION

1. Add 5 ml of saline solution to a nebulizer chamber.
2. Add 3 drops of diluted DMSO and mix gently.
3. Use the nebulizer for 10 minutes.

Safe Dosages and Usage Guidelines: Use once daily for lung hydration.

Turmeric & DMSO Gargle for Throat and Bronchial Support

INGREDIENTS

- Ground turmeric
- DMSO (99% pure, diluted to 30%)
- Warm water

PREPARATION

1. Dissolve 1/2 teaspoon of turmeric in 1/2 cup of warm water.
2. Add 5 drops of diluted DMSO and stir well.
3. Gargle for 30 seconds and spit out.

Safe Dosages and Usage Guidelines: Use once daily for throat and bronchial relief.

Magnesium Oil & DMSO Topical Blend for Respiratory Muscle Relaxation

INGREDIENTS

- Magnesium oil
- DMSO (99% pure, diluted to 50%)

PREPARATION

1. Mix 1 teaspoon of magnesium oil with 5 drops of diluted DMSO.
2. Massage onto the chest and back area.

Safe Dosages and Usage Guidelines: Apply once daily for muscle relaxation.

Ginger & DMSO Warm Compress for Chest Congestion

INGREDIENTS

- Fresh ginger juice
- DMSO (99% pure, diluted to 30%)
- Warm water
- Clean cloth

PREPARATION

1. Mix 1 teaspoon of ginger juice with 5 drops of diluted DMSO.
2. Soak a clean cloth in warm water and wring out excess liquid.
3. Apply the ginger-DMSO mixture to the cloth and place it on the chest for 15 minutes.

Safe Dosages and Usage Guidelines: Use once daily to ease chest congestion.

Licorice Root & DMSO Tonic for Lung Inflammation Control

INGREDIENTS

- Licorice root tea
- DMSO (99% pure, diluted to 30%)

PREPARATION

1. Brew 1 cup of licorice root tea and let it cool slightly.
2. Add 5 drops of diluted DMSO and stir well.

Safe Dosages and Usage Guidelines: Consume once daily to manage lung inflammation.

Aloe Vera & DMSO Drink for Mucosal Lining Protection

INGREDIENTS

- Aloe vera juice
- DMSO (99% pure, diluted to 30%)
- Filtered water

PREPARATION

1. Mix 1 tablespoon of aloe vera juice with 5 drops of diluted DMSO.
2. Add 1/2 cup of filtered water and stir well.

Safe Dosages and Usage Guidelines: Drink once daily for mucosal lining support.

Thyme & DMSO Herbal Infusion for Bronchial Support

INGREDIENTS

- Dried thyme leaves
- DMSO (99% pure, diluted to 30%)
- Hot water

PREPARATION

1. Steep 1 teaspoon of dried thyme leaves in 1 cup of hot water for 10 minutes.
2. Strain and let it cool to lukewarm.
3. Add 5 drops of diluted DMSO and stir.

Safe Dosages and Usage Guidelines: Drink once daily to support bronchial health.

和
BOOK 18
DMSO REMEDIES FOR SURGERY AND RECOVERY (PREVENTING POST-OP INFECTIONS)

CHAPTER 32
POST-SURGICAL HEALING AND INFECTION PREVENTION WITH DMSO

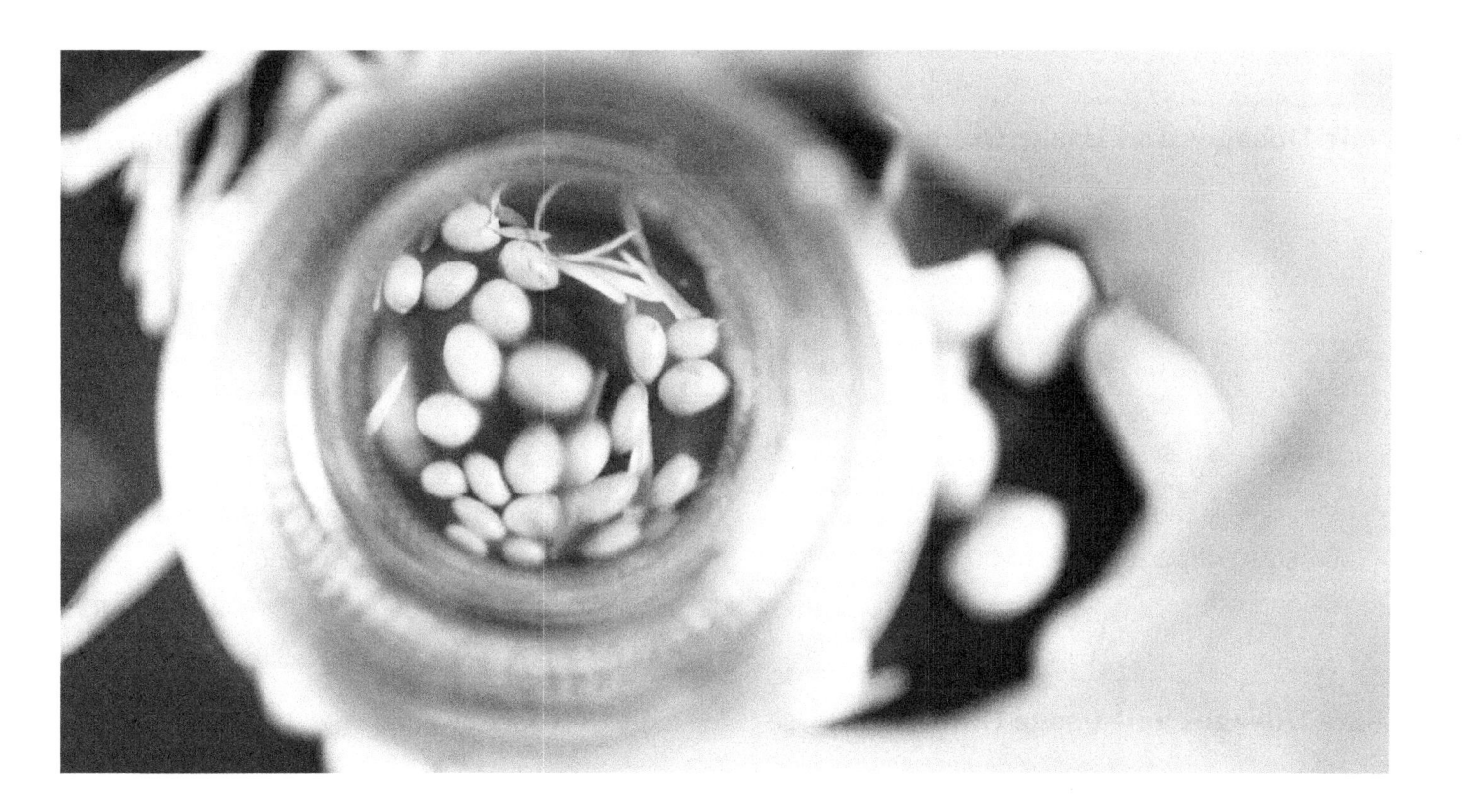

DMSO & Aloe Vera Gel for Scar Reduction and Skin Regeneration

INGREDIENTS

- Aloe vera gel
- DMSO (99% pure, diluted to 50%)

PREPARATION

1. Mix 1 tablespoon of aloe vera gel with 5 drops of diluted DMSO.
2. Apply the mixture directly to the scarred area.
3. Leave it on for at least 15 minutes before rinsing.

Safe Dosages and Usage Guidelines: Apply once daily to reduce scarring and promote skin regeneration.

Honey & DMSO Wound Dressing for Natural Antibacterial Protection

INGREDIENTS

- Raw honey
- DMSO (99% pure, diluted to 30%)

PREPARATION

1. Mix 1 teaspoon of raw honey with 5 drops of diluted DMSO.
2. Spread the mixture onto a sterile gauze pad.
3. Apply the pad to the wound and secure it with a bandage.

Safe Dosages and Usage Guidelines: Change the dressing once daily to prevent infections.

Chamomile & DMSO Compress for Post-Surgical Swelling Control

INGREDIENTS

- Chamomile tea
- DMSO (99% pure, diluted to 30%)
- Clean cloth

PREPARATION

1. Brew 1 cup of chamomile tea and let it cool.
2. Add 5 drops of diluted DMSO and mix.
3. Soak a clean cloth in the solution and apply it to the swollen area.

Safe Dosages and Usage Guidelines: Use twice daily to reduce swelling.

Coconut Oil & DMSO Blend for Skin Hydration and Healing Support

INGREDIENTS

- Coconut oil
- DMSO (99% pure, diluted to 50%)

PREPARATION

1. Mix 1 teaspoon of coconut oil with 5 drops of diluted DMSO.
2. Massage gently onto the skin.

Safe Dosages and Usage Guidelines: Apply once daily to promote hydration and healing.

Collagen & DMSO Topical Solution for Tissue Repair Enhancement

INGREDIENTS

- Collagen powder
- DMSO (99% pure, diluted to 30%)
- Filtered water

PREPARATION

1. Dissolve 1 teaspoon of collagen powder in 2 tablespoons of filtered water.
2. Add 5 drops of diluted DMSO and stir well.
3. Apply the solution directly to the affected area.

Safe Dosages and Usage Guidelines: Use once daily to enhance tissue repair.

Turmeric & DMSO Infused Oil for Reducing Post-Op Inflammation

INGREDIENTS

- Turmeric powder
- Carrier oil (e.g., olive or coconut oil)
- DMSO (99% pure, diluted to 50%)

PREPARATION

1. Mix 1 teaspoon of turmeric powder with 1 tablespoon of carrier oil.
2. Add 5 drops of diluted DMSO and mix well.
3. Apply to the inflamed area.

Safe Dosages and Usage Guidelines: Use once daily to control inflammation.

Saline & DMSO Spray for Gentle Wound Cleansing

INGREDIENTS

- Sterile saline solution
- DMSO (99% pure, diluted to 30%)
- Spray bottle

PREPARATION

1. Fill a spray bottle with 1/2 cup of sterile saline solution.
2. Add 5 drops of diluted DMSO and shake gently.
3. Spray directly onto the wound.

Safe Dosages and Usage Guidelines: Use twice daily for gentle wound cleansing.

MSM & DMSO Lotion for Pain Relief and Recovery Acceleration

INGREDIENTS

- MSM powder
- Unscented lotion
- DMSO (99% pure, diluted to 30%)

PREPARATION

1. Mix 1 teaspoon of MSM powder with 1 tablespoon of unscented lotion.
2. Add 5 drops of diluted DMSO and mix thoroughly.
3. Massage onto the affected area.

Safe Dosages and Usage Guidelines: Apply once daily to reduce pain and accelerate recovery.

Green Tea Extract & DMSO Serum for Skin Soothing and Repair

INGREDIENTS

- Green tea extract
- DMSO (99% pure, diluted to 30%)
- Aloe vera gel

PREPARATION

1. Mix 1 teaspoon of green tea extract with 1 teaspoon of aloe vera gel.
2. Add 5 drops of diluted DMSO and stir well.
3. Apply gently to the skin.

Safe Dosages and Usage Guidelines: Use once daily to soothe and repair skin.

Vitamin E & DMSO Scar Treatment for Enhanced Healing

INGREDIENTS

- Vitamin E oil
- DMSO (99% pure, diluted to 50%)

PREPARATION

1. Mix 1 teaspoon of vitamin E oil with 5 drops of diluted DMSO.
2. Apply to the scarred area using gentle circular motions.

Safe Dosages and Usage Guidelines: Use once daily to enhance scar healing.

BOOK 19

DMSO REMEDIES FOR SYNERGY WITH OXYGEN, MSM, AND NATURAL THERAPIES

CHAPTER 33
ENHANCING DMSO'S EFFECTS WITH NATURAL HEALING COMBINATIONS

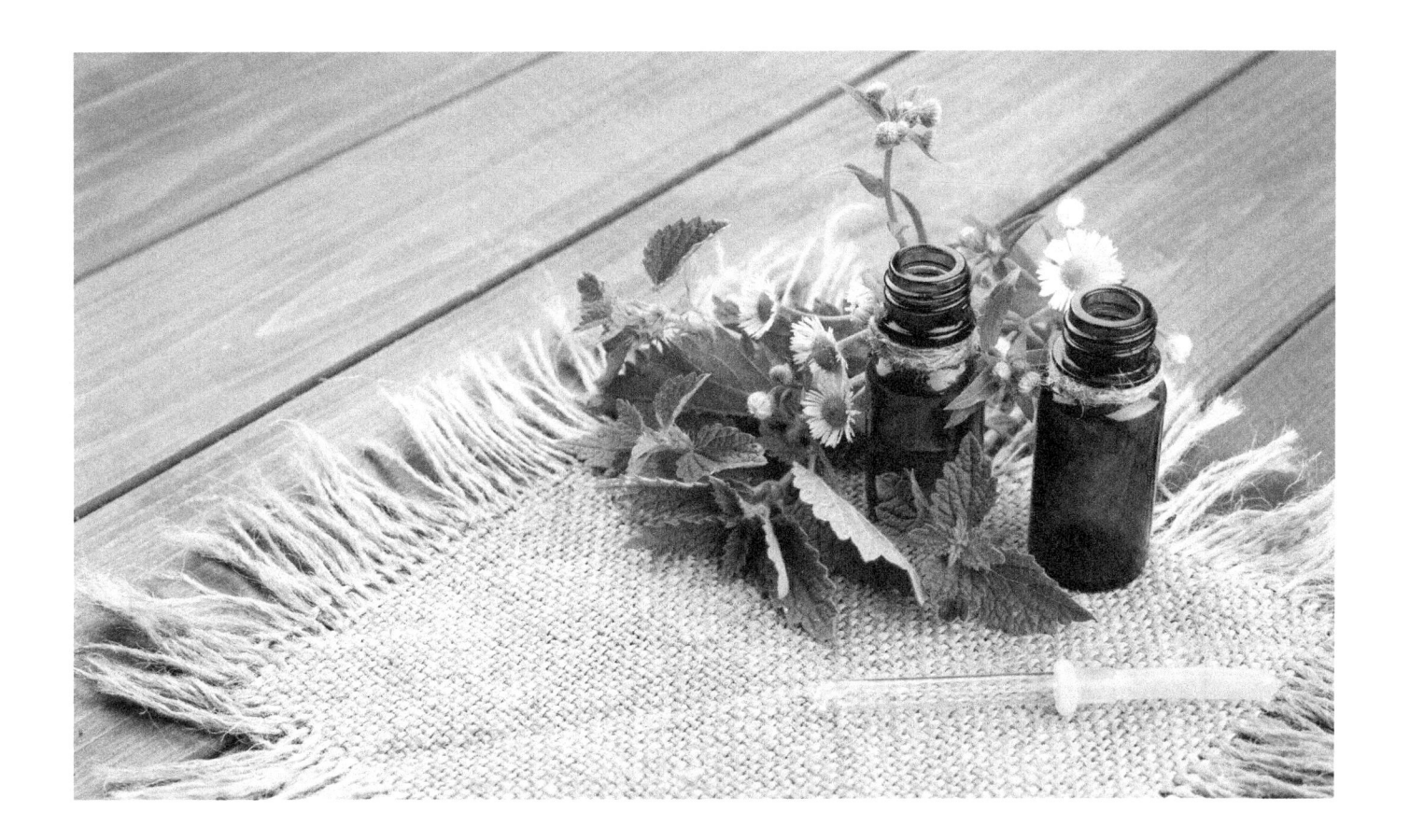

DMSO & MSM Lotion for Joint Flexibility and Pain Relief

INGREDIENTS
- MSM powder
- Unscented lotion
- DMSO (99% pure, diluted to 50%)

PREPARATION
1. Mix 1 teaspoon of MSM powder with 1 tablespoon of unscented lotion.
2. Add 5 drops of diluted DMSO and blend well.
3. Massage onto joints and sore areas.

Safe Dosages and Usage Guidelines: Apply once daily for pain relief and joint flexibility.

Hydrogen Peroxide & DMSO Solution for Skin and Wound Oxygenation

INGREDIENTS

- Food-grade hydrogen peroxide (3%)
- Sterile water
- DMSO (99% pure, diluted to 30%)

PREPARATION

1. Dilute 1 teaspoon of hydrogen peroxide in 1/2 cup of sterile water.
2. Add 5 drops of diluted DMSO and mix gently.
3. Apply with a sterile cotton pad to wounds or skin.

Safe Dosages and Usage Guidelines: Use once daily for wound healing and oxygenation.

Ozone-Infused Olive Oil & DMSO Blend for Antimicrobial Support

INGREDIENTS

- Ozone-infused olive oil
- DMSO (99% pure, diluted to 30%)

PREPARATION

1. Mix 1 teaspoon of ozone-infused olive oil with 5 drops of diluted DMSO.
2. Apply a thin layer to the affected skin.

Safe Dosages and Usage Guidelines: Use once daily for antimicrobial support.

Magnesium & DMSO Spray for Muscle Relaxation and Recovery

INGREDIENTS

- Magnesium oil
- DMSO (99% pure, diluted to 50%)
- Spray bottle

PREPARATION

1. Mix 1/4 cup of magnesium oil with 10 drops of diluted DMSO.
2. Pour into a spray bottle and shake gently.
3. Spray onto sore muscles and massage lightly.

Safe Dosages and Usage Guidelines: Use after exercise or as needed for muscle relaxation.

Coenzyme Q10 & DMSO Topical Application for Cellular Energy Boost

INGREDIENTS

- Coenzyme Q10 liquid extract
- DMSO (99% pure, diluted to 30%)
- Aloe vera gel

PREPARATION

1. Mix 5 drops of coenzyme Q10 extract with 1 teaspoon of aloe vera gel.
2. Add 5 drops of diluted DMSO and blend.
3. Apply to the skin and let absorb.

Safe Dosages and Usage Guidelines: Use once daily for cellular energy support.

Chlorella & DMSO Detox Formula for Heavy Metal Removal

INGREDIENTS

- Chlorella powder
- DMSO (99% pure, diluted to 50%)
- Filtered water

PREPARATION

1. Mix 1 teaspoon of chlorella powder with 1 tablespoon of filtered water.
2. Add 5 drops of diluted DMSO and stir well.
3. Drink immediately.

Safe Dosages and Usage Guidelines: Consume once daily for detox support.

Arnica & DMSO Gel for Bruise and Inflammation Recovery

INGREDIENTS

- Arnica gel
- DMSO (99% pure, diluted to 30%)

PREPARATION

1. Mix 1 teaspoon of arnica gel with 5 drops of diluted DMSO.
2. Apply gently to bruised or swollen areas.

Safe Dosages and Usage Guidelines: Use once daily for inflammation relief.

Omega-3 & DMSO Massage Oil for Cardiovascular and Anti-Inflammatory Benefits

INGREDIENTS

- Omega-3 fish oil
- DMSO (99% pure, diluted to 50%)
- Carrier oil (e.g., coconut or olive oil)

PREPARATION

1. Mix 1 teaspoon of omega-3 fish oil with 1 tablespoon of carrier oil.
2. Add 5 drops of diluted DMSO and blend.
3. Massage onto the skin.

Safe Dosages and Usage Guidelines: Use once daily for cardiovascular support.

Vitamin C & DMSO Serum for Skin Regeneration and Antioxidant Protection

INGREDIENTS

- Vitamin C powder
- Distilled water
- DMSO (99% pure, diluted to 30%)

PREPARATION

1. Dissolve 1 teaspoon of vitamin C powder in 1/2 cup of distilled water.
2. Add 5 drops of diluted DMSO and mix.
3. Apply to the skin using a cotton pad.

Safe Dosages and Usage Guidelines: Use once daily for skin protection and repair.

Ashwagandha & DMSO Adaptogenic Blend for Stress and Immune Support

INGREDIENTS

- Ashwagandha powder
- DMSO (99% pure, diluted to 50%)
- Filtered water

PREPARATION

1. Mix 1 teaspoon of ashwagandha powder with 1/2 cup of filtered water.
2. Add 5 drops of diluted DMSO and stir well.
3. Drink immediately.

Safe Dosages and Usage Guidelines: Take once daily for stress and immune support.

BOOK 20
FINAL THOUGHTS AND PERSONALIZED HEALING PLANS

CHAPTER 34
CUSTOMIZING DMSO TREATMENTS FOR INDIVIDUAL NEEDS

How to Create Your Own Protocols

When it comes to DMSO therapy, no single approach fits everyone. The versatility of DMSO allows for personalized protocols, tailored to an individual's specific condition, lifestyle, and response to treatment. Understanding how to create a customized protocol ensures safe, effective, and targeted use.

Determining the Right Application Method

The method of application depends on the intended purpose and the severity of the condition being treated. There are several ways to use DMSO, each with its own advantages:

- **Topical Application:** The most common method, suitable for pain relief, inflammation, skin conditions, and injuries. Applied directly to the skin, it penetrates tissues rapidly and can carry other substances into the bloodstream.
- **Diluted DMSO for Sensitive Areas:** Certain areas, such as the face, joints, or delicate skin, may require a lower concentration to avoid irritation.
- **Oral Use:** Some protocols involve diluted DMSO solutions for internal detoxification and systemic effects. However, this method requires careful dilution and professional guidance.
- **Nebulized DMSO:** Used for respiratory conditions like asthma or COPD, DMSO can be inhaled when properly diluted with sterile saline. This should be done under expert supervision.
- **Combination Therapy:** DMSO is often paired with complementary treatments, such as herbal extracts, MSM, or vitamin C, to enhance its therapeutic effects.

Choosing the Right Concentration

DMSO is highly potent, and different conditions require different dilution levels to balance effectiveness with safety. The right concentration depends on skin sensitivity, treatment frequency, and location of application.

- **50-70% DMSO:** Used for chronic pain, arthritis, deep inflammation, and muscle recovery.
- **30-50% DMSO:** Suitable for regular use, particularly for joint issues and injuries.
- **10-20% DMSO:** Recommended for facial applications, delicate skin, and nerve-related conditions.

Setting Treatment Frequency and Duration

Customizing a DMSO protocol requires an understanding of dosing intervals to avoid overuse while maximizing benefits.

- **Acute Conditions:** In cases of injuries, sprains, or sudden inflammation, DMSO can be applied 2-3 times per day for the first few days, then reduced as symptoms improve.
- **Chronic Conditions:** For long-term issues like arthritis, neuropathy, or autoimmune conditions, DMSO is often used once or twice daily over extended periods.
- **Maintenance Protocols:** For general wellness or preventive care, lower concentrations applied a few times per week may be sufficient.

Monitoring for Sensitivity and Reactions

Since each individual reacts differently, it's important to monitor the body's response when starting a new protocol. Signs that a protocol adjustment may be needed include:

- **Skin irritation or redness:** A sign that the concentration is too strong for the treated area.
- **Garlic-like odor on breath or skin:** A normal effect of DMSO metabolism but may indicate a need for lower doses.
- **Mild detox symptoms:** Some users experience headaches, fatigue, or digestive changes as toxins are flushed from the system.

Adjusting the dosage or frequency can help the body adapt more smoothly to the treatment.

Combining DMSO with Other Natural Compounds

DMSO works synergistically with many natural anti-inflammatory and healing compounds. Some common combinations include:

- **MSM (Methylsulfonylmethane):** Enhances joint support and helps reduce inflammation.
- **Vitamin C:** Supports immune function and helps neutralize oxidative stress.
- **Turmeric/Curcumin:** Adds anti-inflammatory properties and supports joint health.
- **Aloe Vera or Magnesium Oil:** Helps soothe skin when used in topical blends.

Tracking Progress and Adjusting Over Time

Because DMSO is a dynamic compound, regular adjustments may be needed based on how the body responds. Keeping a treatment log can help users identify patterns, track improvements, and fine-tune their approach.

By following these principles, individuals can develop personalized DMSO protocols that align with their unique health needs, ensuring safe and effective use.

Adjusting Dosages Based on Health Conditions

When using DMSO therapeutically, proper dosing is critical to achieve the desired effects while minimizing the risk of side effects. Because each individual reacts differently, dosages must be adjusted based on the condition being treated, the sensitivity of the user, and the method of application. Understanding how to tailor DMSO concentrations and frequency ensures safe and effective use across a range of health conditions.

Factors That Influence Dosage Adjustments

DMSO dosages are not one-size-fits-all. Several key factors determine the appropriate strength and frequency:

- **Severity of the condition:** Chronic conditions often require lower doses over extended periods, while acute conditions may benefit from higher concentrations for short-term use.
- **Area of application:** Sensitive areas such as the face, joints, or mucous membranes require lower concentrations to prevent irritation.
- **Individual sensitivity:** Some individuals may be more prone to skin irritation, detox reactions, or strong metabolic responses, requiring gradual dose adjustments.
- **Combination with other therapies:** DMSO's ability to enhance the absorption of other substances means that dosages should be adjusted when used alongside medications, supplements, or alternative treatments.

Dosage Guidelines for Specific Conditions

Each health condition requires a different approach to DMSO dosing. Adjusting dosages based on the type of issue being addressed ensures optimal benefits while minimizing risks.

Joint Pain and Arthritis

For arthritis, tendonitis, and inflammatory joint conditions, DMSO is typically used topically to reduce pain and inflammation.

- **Concentration:** 50-70% DMSO, applied directly to affected joints.
- **Frequency:** 1-2 times daily for chronic pain; up to 3 times daily for acute flare-ups.
- **Adjustment considerations:** If irritation occurs, diluting to 30-50% may be necessary.

Neuropathy and Nerve Damage

DMSO helps stimulate nerve repair and reduce neuropathic pain. However, nerves are highly sensitive, so concentration must be carefully controlled.

- **Concentration:** 25-50% DMSO, depending on skin sensitivity.
- **Frequency:** Once daily for chronic conditions; twice daily for more severe cases.

- **Adjustment considerations:** Higher concentrations may cause tingling or temporary discomfort; reducing to 20-30% can help.

Autoimmune Conditions

For conditions like lupus, fibromyalgia, or multiple sclerosis, DMSO is often used systemically to reduce inflammation and immune overactivity.

- **Concentration:** 25-50% DMSO, applied topically or used in diluted oral protocols (under medical supervision).
- **Frequency:** Once daily, with careful monitoring for detox symptoms.
- **Adjustment considerations:** Some individuals may experience fatigue or detox reactions, requiring lower concentrations or less frequent use.

Sports Injuries and Muscle Recovery

DMSO accelerates healing of sprains, strains, and muscle soreness.

- **Concentration:** 50-70% DMSO, applied over the affected area.
- **Frequency:** 2-3 times daily for acute injuries, once daily for recovery maintenance.
- **Adjustment considerations:** Lower concentrations may be needed for sensitive skin areas to prevent irritation.

Detoxification and Heavy Metal Removal

DMSO supports detoxification by binding to toxins and promoting their elimination.

- **Concentration:** 30-50% DMSO, applied topically or used in low-dose oral regimens (under guidance).
- **Frequency:** Every other day to prevent detox overload.
- **Adjustment considerations:** Some users experience headaches or fatigue as toxins are released; reducing frequency or concentration can help manage symptoms.

Gradual Dose Adjustments for Safety

Because DMSO is highly potent, making gradual adjustments helps the body adapt without unwanted side effects.

- Start with a lower concentration and increase as needed.
- Monitor for side effects like skin irritation, detox reactions, or mild fatigue.
- Space out treatments if reactions occur, allowing the body to adjust.
- Consider rotating application areas to prevent skin sensitivity.

By customizing dosages based on health conditions, individuals can safely harness DMSO's full therapeutic potential while minimizing risks and ensuring long-term benefits.

CHAPTER 35
THE FUTURE OF DMSO IN NATURAL MEDICINE

Emerging Research and New Applications

As DMSO continues to gain recognition in alternative medicine, researchers are exploring new therapeutic applications that extend beyond its well-established uses. While its ability to reduce inflammation, enhance drug absorption, and support cellular repair is well-documented, modern scientific inquiry is uncovering even more potential benefits. These emerging areas of research pave the way for DMSO's future integration into holistic and conventional medicine.

DMSO and Stem Cell Therapy

One of the most exciting developments in DMSO research is its potential synergy with stem cell therapy. Scientists are investigating how DMSO can:

- Preserve and protect stem cells during transplantation.
- Enhance the differentiation of stem cells into functional tissues.
- Reduce inflammation that could interfere with successful cell integration.

This research suggests that DMSO may increase the success rate of regenerative medicine techniques, particularly in treating neurodegenerative diseases, joint disorders, and spinal cord injuries.

DMSO's Role in Cardiovascular Health

Another area of emerging interest is DMSO's impact on cardiovascular function. Studies indicate that it may:

- Improve blood flow and circulation by reducing clot formation.
- Reduce oxidative stress in blood vessels, helping to lower hypertension risk.
- Aid in post-stroke recovery by minimizing damage from ischemia.

These findings suggest that DMSO may have potential therapeutic applications for individuals with heart disease, poor circulation, and vascular inflammation.

DMSO and Cancer Research

While DMSO's role in cancer support has been controversial, new studies explore how it may:

- Enhance the effectiveness of chemotherapy drugs while reducing their toxicity.
- Improve cellular oxygenation, a factor that may help in inhibiting tumor growth.
- Support the immune system's ability to target abnormal cells.

Although further clinical trials are needed, researchers are exploring DMSO's integration into integrative cancer care protocols.

DMSO for Brain and Neurological Health

Emerging research is also pointing to DMSO's neuroprotective properties. Studies suggest that it can:

- Cross the blood-brain barrier, delivering anti-inflammatory compounds directly to the brain.
- Reduce neuroinflammation, potentially benefiting conditions like Alzheimer's, multiple sclerosis, and traumatic brain injuries.
- Support mitochondrial function, which is crucial for preventing neurodegenerative diseases.

These findings indicate that DMSO may play a role in long-term brain health and cognitive function.

Expanding Topical and Internal Uses

As scientists continue to investigate DMSO's bioavailability and mechanism of action, new topical and systemic applications are being explored, including:

- Transdermal patches for pain management and targeted drug delivery.
- Low-dose oral formulations for immune modulation and gut health.
- Combination therapies with herbal and nutraceutical compounds for enhanced healing.

As research advances, DMSO is likely to become an even more versatile tool in holistic medicine, expanding its applications for disease prevention, recovery, and cellular regeneration.

How to Safely Integrate DMSO Into a Holistic Health Plan

Integrating DMSO into a holistic health regimen requires careful consideration, proper dosing, and a well-structured plan that complements other natural therapies. While DMSO offers exceptional healing properties, its effectiveness depends on how it is used, combined with other treatments, and incorporated into daily wellness practices. A well-rounded approach ensures optimal benefits while minimizing risks.

Understanding the Synergy of DMSO with Other Natural Therapies

DMSO is most effective when combined with other holistic modalities that enhance its therapeutic effects. Some key elements to consider when integrating DMSO into a natural health plan include:

- **Anti-inflammatory nutrition:** A diet rich in whole foods, healthy fats, and antioxidants enhances DMSO's ability to reduce inflammation at a cellular level.
- **Detoxification support:** Incorporating liver-supportive herbs, hydration, and gentle detox strategies may help the body process toxins that DMSO mobilizes.
- **Complementary therapies:** DMSO can be synergistic with ozone therapy, herbal medicine, and vitamin supplementation, further amplifying its benefits.
- **Mind-body balance:** Stress management techniques such as meditation, deep breathing, and light exercise contribute to enhanced cellular recovery when using DMSO.

Determining the Right Dosage for Individual Needs

DMSO is not a one-size-fits-all treatment, and individual health conditions, sensitivity levels, and treatment goals all play a role in dosage selection. A safe approach involves:

- **Starting with low concentrations:** Many individuals begin with a diluted form of DMSO (typically 50-70%) to assess tolerance and avoid skin irritation.
- **Observing body responses:** Monitoring for any discomfort, detox reactions, or sensitivities is essential to adjusting the regimen accordingly.
- **Considering frequency and duration:** Short-term usage for acute inflammation differs from long-term protocols for chronic conditions. Adjusting based on progress and symptoms is crucial.
- **Avoiding overuse:** More is not always better—excessive use can overwhelm the body's detox pathways and lead to unwanted side effects.

Safe Application Methods for Maximum Effectiveness

Since DMSO rapidly penetrates tissues, handling it correctly is key to ensuring both safety and efficacy. Important precautions include:

- Using only pharmaceutical-grade DMSO to avoid contamination with industrial solvents.
- Applying with clean hands and tools to prevent the absorption of unwanted chemicals into the bloodstream.
- Diluting appropriately when applying topically to prevent skin irritation or burning.
- Avoiding synthetic fabrics after application, as DMSO can carry fabric chemicals into the body.

Customizing DMSO Protocols for Long-Term Wellness

For individuals seeking long-term benefits, DMSO can be integrated into a personalized health plan based on specific wellness goals. Some key factors in designing a sustainable protocol include:

- **Cycling usage:** Alternating periods of use and rest allows the body to adapt and recover.

- **Targeting different systems:** Whether supporting joint health, neurological function, or detoxification, adjusting formulations and application areas can optimize results.
- **Pairing with hydration and mineral balance:** Since DMSO can influence fluid balance, ensuring adequate hydration and electrolyte intake is critical.

By integrating DMSO mindfully and strategically, it becomes a powerful tool in holistic healing, enhancing the body's natural regenerative processes while supporting overall well-being.

Medical Disclaimer

This book is intended for informational and educational purposes only. The content provided herein is not meant to diagnose, treat, cure, or prevent any disease. The use of DMSO or any other remedy mentioned in this book should not be considered a substitute for professional medical advice, diagnosis, or treatment.

Always consult a qualified healthcare professional before using DMSO or making any changes to your health regimen, especially if you have pre-existing conditions, are pregnant, nursing, or taking medications. The authors and publishers assume no responsibility for any adverse effects resulting from the application of the information contained in this book.

By choosing to use any of the remedies or protocols mentioned, the reader acknowledges and accepts full responsibility for their health decisions.

YOUR EXCLUSIVE BONUS

Scan the QR-CODE below to get your exclusive bonus!

Made in the USA
Columbia, SC
24 July 2025